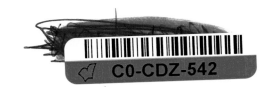

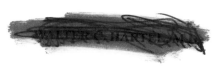

NUCLEAR MAGNETIC RESONANCE IMAGING
Basic Principles

Nuclear Magnetic Resonance Imaging

Basic Principles

Stuart W. Young, M.D.

Department of Diagnostic Radiology
Stanford University Medical Center
Stanford, California

Raven Press ■ New York

Raven Press, 1140 Avenue of the Americas, New York, New York 10036

Library of Congress Cataloging in Publication Data

Young, Stuart W.
  Nuclear magnetic resonance imaging.

  Bibliography: p.
  Includes index.
  1. Nuclear magnetic resonance—Diagnostic use.
2. Imaging systems in medicine. I. Title.
RC78.7.N83Y68 1984   616.07′575   83-42621
ISBN 0-89004-998-X

Made in the United States of America

Great care has been taken to maintain the accuracy of the information contained in the volume. However, Raven Press cannot be held responsible for errors or for any consequences arising from the use of the information contained herein.

Second Printing, July 1984

To Susan

Preface

This book has been organized to give an overview of the clinical and biological potential of nuclear magnetic resonance (NMR) imaging, and then proceeds to discuss the fundamental principles of the interaction of NMR and electromagnetic waves to generate the NMR signal on which NMR images are based. Subsequently, the components of the NMR signal, i.e., proton density, relaxation times (T_1 and T_2), and motion or flow, are introduced together with their various interpretations and effects on image contrast.

Finally, some of the potential applications of NMR are introduced as well as the types of current imaging systems available. The book concludes with a chapter that considers the hazards of NMR imaging and site planning, as well as a reference section for those desiring to do further reading in this area.

NMR imaging in all likelihood will become increasingly more important to a broad spectrum of health professionals and investigators. This book has been compiled so that a broad spectrum of readers with general imaging or NMR background or biological and physiological medical backgrounds will be able to understand the basic principles of NMR imaging and gain enough background to progress to more in-depth NMR studies in their respective medical subspecialties. Health professionals who have been previously concerned with imaging subspecialties will benefit from becoming familiar with the physical principles of NMR, and those who have a background in NMR will further gain from the sections that are devoted to imaging and anatomic correlation. Finally, other health professionals without background in imaging or NMR should find the principles, as illustrated by analogies from common experience, helpful in understanding this complex technology.

Stuart W. Young

Acknowledgments

I am indebted to Albert Macovski, Ph.D., C. Leon Partain, Ph.D., M.D., Oleg Jardetzky, M.D., Ph.D., Ronald Castellino, M.D., Leslie M. Zatz, M.D., and Dieter Enzmann, M.D. for critical review of the manuscript. I am deeply indebted to Mike Mesenbrink, University Hospitals of Cleveland, Ralph Alfidi, M.D., Cleveland Clinic Foundation, Thomas Meaney, M.D., Mickey Weinstein, M.D. and Technicare Corporation; Felix Wehrli, Ph.D. and Morry Blumenfeld, Ph.D. The Medical College of Wisconsin and the General Electric Company; Michael Brant-Zawadski, M.D. and Leon Kaufman, Ph.D., Radiologic Imaging Laboratory, University of California, San Francisco; and Raymond Damadian and Fonar, Incorporated; for permission to utilize the NMR figures presented in this book. The author gratefully acknowledges the invaluable assistance of Charlene Levering and the Medical Graphics staff of Stanford's Office of Instructual Media for their patient work in preparing the graphic illustrations. This is the first text to be done completely by computer graphics. My thanks to Marie Graham and Lynn Roussell for manuscript preparation and word processing. And finally I am indebted to William Bradley, M.D., Ph.D. and Don Plewis, Ph.D. for general background illustrations on the physics and principles of NMR imaging.

Foreword

Nuclear magnetic resonance (NMR), long an established powerful research tool of the physicist, chemist, and molecular biologist has finally caught the imagination of the practicing clinician as a noninvasive technique for medical diagnosis that has an unprecedented wealth of information, versatility, and potential in medicine. The successful combination of NMR spectroscopy with established image reconstruction techniques, pioneered by Paul Lauterbur, and the construction of stable high resolution magnets with bores large enough to accommodate the human body during the past decade have provided the main impetus for this development. With it arose the need for an introductory text on NMR and its potential medical applications for the clinician who until now had little reason to worry about the intricacies of exotic physical techniques.

Dr. Young has written a lucid introduction to the fundamentals of NMR, relating by many imaginative analogies the physical principles of the method to similar physical phenomena more familiar from everyday life. Mastery of these concepts will be indispensable not only to the researcher, but to the clinical diagnostician as well. NMR is inherently a more complicated physical phenomenon than the scattering of X-rays. As a result, a greater variety of information can be extracted from NMR observations, but there is also a far greater danger of misinterpretation and instrumental artifact. Purely empirical correlations may prove treacherous, because of the larger number of physical variables involved. To be confident of a diagnostic finding we will need to have not just density, as in X-rays, but also the chemical shift, T1, T2, and RF pulse sequences as part of our second nature. The reader of this book will be well on the way to absorbing them into his intuitive armamentarium.

Whether we enter this new field with expertise in NMR or in clinical medicine, we must however remember that we are all still beginners. We have learned how to measure chemical shifts, T1 and T2 in living systems, and we are rapidly learning how differences in these variables affect the images and the measurements we make, but we have very little understanding of the factors that determine them in normal and diseased tissues. We understand the physics, but almost not at all the chemistry of what we see. It is the access to chemical information, both in the imaging and in the spectroscopic mode that makes NMR uniquely versatile among the existing research and diagnostic methods. Therein lies the great challenge to the experimentalist and the clinician. We should meet this challenge with vigor, but also with caution, aware that we are standing before a virtually untapped treasure of new information, but also always bearing in mind that a little knowledge can be a dangerous thing.

Oleg Jardetzky

Contents

Chapter 1

Nuclear Magnetic Resonance: The Clinical Potential

Magnetic resonance medical imaging is becoming very important in the clinical management of patients. The information density in the nuclear magnetic resonance (NMR) signal is greater than that available in an imaging modality like computed tomography (X-ray CT) because the magnetic resonance signal is based on four separate components: density of the nuclear species (usually hydrogen, which is composed of a single proton—^{1}H), two relaxation times (T_1 and T_2), and motion or flow. The computed tomography (X-ray CT) radiographic image, by comparison, is based mainly on one tissue characteristic: electron density. The information available in nuclear magnetic resonance (NMR) images will in all likelihood be further enriched when other nuclear species such as phosphorus and carbon can be scanned in clinical NMR scanners. The signals from nuclear species other than ^{1}H are low, and therefore, the likely format will be to superimpose phosphorus or carbon images or spectra on hydrogen density images either by color tinting of the hydrogen image or by superimposing a black dot distribution format similar to autoradiography. Another aspect of NMR imaging that will encourage its clinical utilization is that magnetic resonance imaging does not use ionizing radiation and thus is free of the potential hazards of X-ray interaction with tissue.

The practicing physician, whether an imaging specialist or primary-care physician, may never have encountered NMR imaging and may have previously considered NMR as merely a chemical phenomenon useful for sophisticated chemical analysis. The principles of NMR were actually first described in 1946, and NMR imaging has been used since 1973. Although clinical medical applications of these imaging techniques have only recently been reported, NMR imaging has already been shown to be clearly superior to other competitive

1

imaging modalities (e.g., CT scanning) in certain specific situations. NMR scans are free from the artifacts produced in CT scans by sharp dense bone or metallic surgical clips (i.e., aliasing and overrange artifacts). NMR is the imaging modality of choice in diagnosing multiple sclerosis, and by selecting the proper NMR imaging techniques, in determining accurately areas of edema and hemorrhage which are difficult to separate by X-ray CT. Whether a nodular density in the lung hilum is a normal pulmonary blood vessel or an abnormal tumor mass is a difficult clinical problem with CT scanning or conventional radiography; however, in NMR imaging no signal is returned from rapidly flowing blood, and a very strong signal is returned from benign or neoplastic masses. Thus, this specific clinical problem is easily resolved using NMR. Gated NMR scans appear to be excellent for imaging the myocardium because the flowing blood in the ventricle (no NMR signal) accurately outlines the cardiac muscle. At first glance NMR scans appear very much like CT scans, but there are very definite differences, as illustrated in Figs. 1.1 through 1.8. (CT/NMR scans). A careful examination reveals that the circular high-density region is the bony skull and calvarium on the CT scan with little of the subcutaneous fat and scalp tissue in evidence. However, in the NMR scan the high-density (white) ring structure corresponds to the subcutaneous fat and the bone is seen as a relatively dark or black ring inside the outer white ring of fat. Some white and gray areas within the black ring of the skull indicate the bone marrow, which has a relatively high fat content, and therefore a larger NMR signal than surrounding bone. The comparisons and contrasts between NMR and CT imaging will be expanded in the ensuing chapters.

The tempo of change in medical imaging has been accelerating, and it is continuing to accelerate at a bewildering rate even for those whose expertise is primarily in the imaging sciences. If we borrow a bit of imagery from Carl Sagan and create an imaging calendar to relate chronologically the major breakthroughs in imaging as Sagan related the major events in the development of the cosmos on a galactic calendar, spanning the events from the last big bang to the present, we find our ''imaging big bang'' occurs with the discovery of the roentgen ray by Wilhelm Conrad Röntgen in 1895 (Fig. 1.9). We can see that January in this imaging calendar year was truly a big bang with fluoroscopy, X-ray tubes and X-ray films, all developed in those early stages. Everything else through September of this year was really just a variation on a theme, which required a slightly different application of previously well-understood principles. How-

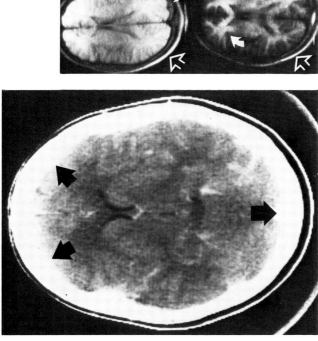

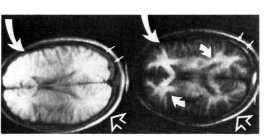

FIG. 1.1. A normal X-ray CT scan (*left*) and a normal NMR scan (*right*) using two different NMR imaging techniques, saturation-recovery (*top*) and inversion-recovery (*bottom*), obtained at the level of the lateral ventricles. Note that on the X-ray CT scan the bone of the skull is a dense white outer ring (*black arrows*) and little of the subcutaneous tissues are visualized, whereas in the NMR scan the bone is noted by its appearance as a black density around the brain (*curved arrows*) and the subcutaneous fat is seen as a dense white circumferential ring (*open white arrows*). Note also that some NMR signal is obtained from the central portion of the bony skull and this signal emanates from the fat contained in the bone marrow (*short arrows*). Also note that by changing the technique of obtaining the NMR image, different features of the tissue can be elucidated. For example, note the improvement in gray-white matter contrast resolution seen on the lower NMR image (inversion-recovery image). In this image white matter (*curved arrowheads*) appears as dense white stellate bands surrounding the lateral ventricles (3 KG, 1-cm slice thickness). (Copyright Technicare Corporation. NMR image provided by courtesy of Technicare Corporation.)

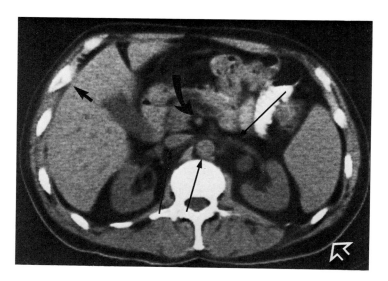

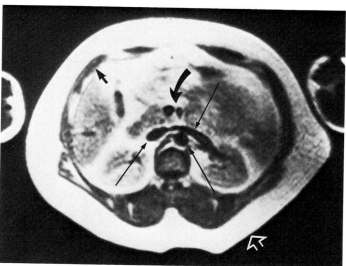

FIG. 1.2. A normal X-ray CT scan (*top*) and a normal NMR scan (*bottom*) obtained at the level of the left renal vein. As in Fig. 1.1, note the reversal in gray scale density between bone, which is white on the X-ray CT scan and black on the NMR scan (*black arrowheads*), and fat, which is black on the X-ray CT scan and white on the NMR scan (*opened white arrows*). Another interesting difference between X-ray CT and NMR scans illustrated by these body sections is the absence of NMR signal obtained from the blood vessels in the NMR scan as opposed to the soft tissue density seen on the X-ray CT scans. This absence of signal especially when juxtaposed with the high-contrast NMR signal from the fat makes the left renal vein, vena cava, and aorta (*long straight arrows*) very easy to identify as well as the superior mesenteric artery and vein (*curved arrows*). The reason for the lack of NMR signal from blood vessels is due to the absence of signal from moving structures in general (3 KG, 1-cm slice thickness). (Copyright Technicare Corporation. NMR image provided by courtesy of Technicare Corporation.)

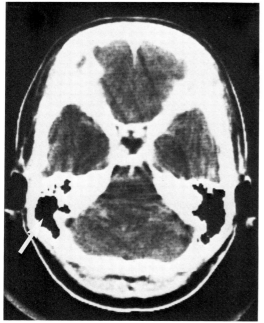
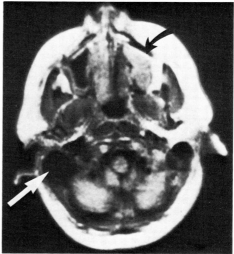

FIG. 1.3. A normal X-ray CT scan (*left*) and a normal NMR scan of the posterior fossa (*right*). Note the white streak artifacts on the CT scan, produced by the dense bone of the posterior fossa, and the absence of these artifacts on the NMR scan. No signal is obtained from the mastoid sinuses in either study (*straight arrow*), and also note opacification of the left maxillary sinus on the NMR scan due to sinusitis (*curved arrow*). (Copyright Technicare Corporation. NMR image provided by courtesy of Technicare Corporation.)

ever, in November things began to pick up with CT imaging, and an imaging "mini-bang" really exploded in December with clinical NMR imaging, digital imaging, digital subtraction angiography (DSA), laser imaging, and medical holography.

HOW TO USE THIS BOOK

For many imaging specialists who have recently become familiar with the principles, techniques, normal anatomy, and artifacts of ultrasound, CT, and digital imaging, the prospect of learning the underlying physical principles and clinical use of an entirely new technology is not considered lightly. There are always those individuals within the imaging community who take the 747 approach in the belief that you do not have to know an aileron from a gyroscope to use the

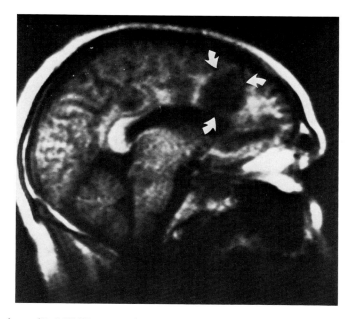

FIG. 1.4. A sagittal NMR scan of a patient with large plaques of multiple scle-rosis, one of which is seen in the frontal lobe (*arrows*) as a low-density lesion on this inversion-recovery image (3 KG, 1-cm slice thickness). (NMR image provided by courtesy of Technicare Corporation and the University Hospitals of Cleveland.)

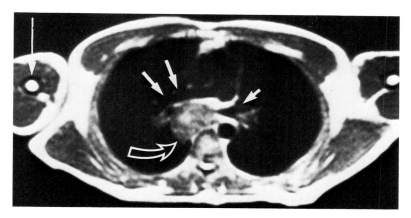

FIG. 1.5. An NMR scan at the level of the hilum demonstrating a large NMR signal from the metastatic carcinoma mass (*open arrow*) that is clearly seen as separate from the blood vessels in the same cut that are only seen because of the absence of NMR signal (*straight arrows*). Note also the bone marrow (*white*) in the humerus and cortical bone surrounding (*black ring, long arrow*) (3 KG, 1-cm slice thickness). (Copyright Technicare Corporation. NMR image provided by courtesy of Technicare Corporation and the University Hospitals of Cleve-land.)

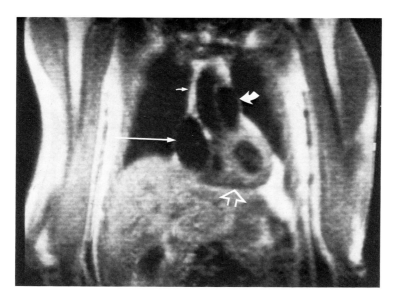

FIG. 1.6. A gated coronal NMR scan illustrating well the left ventricle (*open arrow*) as distinct from the black (lack of NMR signal) intraventricular blood and surrounding lung and fat (*white*) at the apex. Note also in this image the right atrium (*long arrow*), aorta (*short arrow*), pulmonary artery (*curved arrow*), and the proximal humerus with black cortical bone and white marrow (3 KG, 1-cm slice thickness). (Copyright Technicare Corporation. NMR image provided by courtesy of Technicare Corporation.)

747 to get from San Francisco to New York. Nevertheless, NMR will be a very important tool in medical imaging and in all likelihood will at some point exceed CT scanning as a diagnostic modality. To use these techniques, the clinician is consequently obliged to understand the basics of NMR image formation, particularly as it relates to clinical interpretation. To the clinician, magnetic resonance may seem exceptionally complex upon first encounter. However, it is the objective of this book to develop each principle and concept of NMR as if it were a fugue, using many examples from common experience. Each principle will be discussed first, by analogy with sound waves, and second, by analogy with magnetic compass needles. Finally, these analogies will be used as a foundation for the more complex explanations of NMR physics and imaging principles.

Readers of this book will undoubtedly have varying degrees of expertise and experience with magnetic resonance. Many will not need all of the fundamental analogies presented here or may wish to read the explanations in classical physics and quantum mechanics, referring to the analogies only where their understanding is somewhat

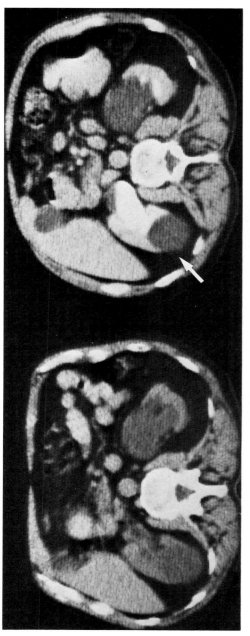

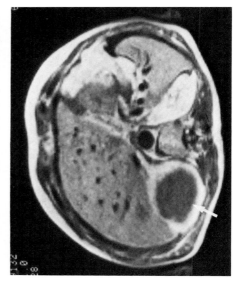

FIG. 1.7.

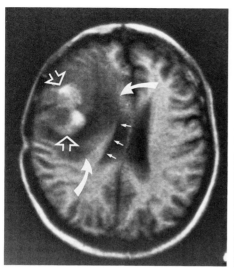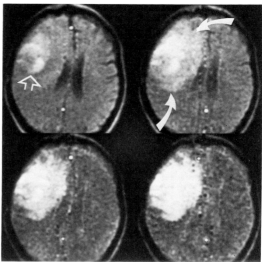

FIG. 1.8. Regions of differing NMR intensity can be discerned in this image of a patient with a recurrent ganglioglioma in the right temporal lobe, recorded by the inversion-recovery technique with a repetition time of 1 sec and an interpulse delay of 500 msec (*left*). Necrotic tissue, due to its somewhat shortened T_1, exhibits enhanced intensity (*open arrows*), whereas tumorous tissue with relative prolongation of T_1, appears as hypointense areas (*curved arrows*). Note compression of lateral ventricle (*arrowheads*).

Using a different imaging sequence called spin-echo (see Chapter 6) multiple echo images obtained with echo delays of 12 to 51 msec (*right—top, left to right*) from the same patient. Note that at an echo delay of 12 msec, primarily necrotic tissue is highlighted, due to its short T_1 (*open arrows*). At 25.5 msec, however, tumorous and edematous tissue, because of prolonged T_2, shows enhanced intensity (*curved arrows*), clearly standing out from the surrounding normal tissue. In the two bottom images (third and fourth echo), on the other hand, the pathologic tissues merge and thus become indistinguishable. Because of the decreased overall signal-to-noise ratio of the higher order echos, the resulting images become progressively noisier. (Copyright General Electric Company. NMR image provided by courtesy of the General Electric Company and the Medical College of Wisconsin.)

FIG. 1.7. An X-ray CT scan obtained before and after (*top*) intravenous contrast media in a patient with a right upper pole renal cyst (*arrow*) and left hydronephrosis, and an NMR scan of a patient with a right upper pole renal cyst (*bottom*). Note that although the right renal cyst is as well defined as the one on the post-contrast X-ray CT scan, it required the administration of intravenous contrast media with its attendant risks to bring the contrast enhancement level up to that seen with the NMR scan (*bottom*) but without the use of any intravenous contrast media (*arrow*). Note the dark circles in the liver that are the portal and hepatic blood vessels (3 KG, 0.5-cm slice thickness). (NMR image courtesy of the University of California San Francisco Radiologic Imaging Laboratory.)

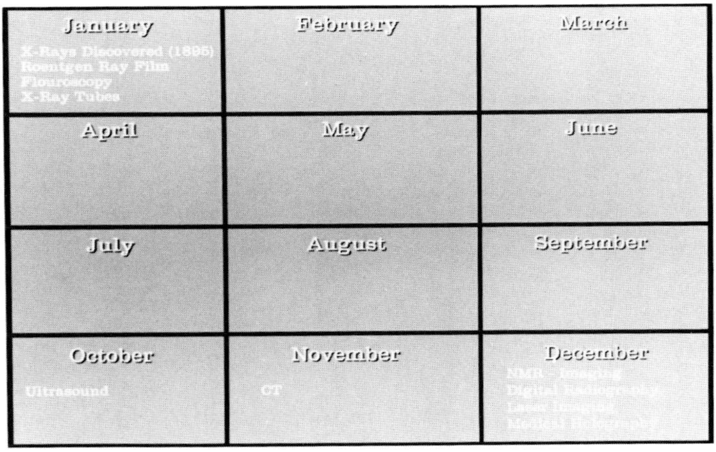

January	February	March
X-Rays Discovered (1895) Roentgen Ray Film Flouroscopy X-Ray Tubes		
April	May	June
July	August	September
October	November	December
Ultrasound	CT	NMR - Imaging Digital Radiography Laser Imaging Medical Holography

FIG. 1.9. The imaging calendar year, if constructed from the time of the discovery of the roentgen ray in 1895, reveals that much of what has occurred since that time has really been refinement and variation on basic radiographic principles and techniques. However, a second nearly overwhelming explosion in imaging technology has recently occurred with the imaging techniques of CT, digital radiography, laser imaging, and NMR scanning.

shaky. Redundancies in the analogies used are purposely included. I have introduced principles as a foundation and subsequently reiterated and built upon them with the hope that concepts not completely comprehensible in one form of imagery will be understandable in another. An NMR quiz is included at the end of this book for those who may wish to evaluate their level of understanding and earmark sections to be included in a quick review of this subject.

Chapter 2

Nuclear Magnetic Resonance: What is it?

The NMR phenomenon was originally described at Stanford by Block and at Harvard by Purcell in 1946. They later received the Nobel prize in 1952 for their work. Briefly, NMR imaging is a way of making pictures of the body that look somewhat like CT scans. Atoms in the body can act like tiny bar magnets with a north and south pole. When an external magnetic field is applied across a part of the body, each little magnet lines up with the external magnetic field. If a radio wave is then broadcast into the body tissue, some of the magnets absorb some of the energy from the radio wave's energy and tilt over. The radio wave is then turned off, and subsequently the magnets rebroadcast the signal they absorbed. This rebroadcasted signal can be picked up by an antenna, and then a computer can make a picture (scan) from the signal.

At this point we shall expand somewhat on this basic definition. However, all of these principles will be discussed in more detail in later sections. In most substances, including living tissues, some of the nuclei within the specimen act as tiny magnets when the specimen is placed in a stable magnetic field. For instance, if you were to place the north and south poles of a bar magnet around your index finger, these nuclear magnets (proton nuclei of hydrogen atoms, ^{1}H) would orient themselves either parallel or antiparallel to that magnetic field, with the antiparallel protons having a slightly higher energy level than the parallel atoms. When the antiparallel atoms give up energy and switch to a parallel relationship with the external magnetic field, the energy is lost in the form of radio waves. These radio waves exit from your finger and can be picked up by any suitable antenna similar to the one on an AM-FM radio. In a static magnetic field the energy emitted from a given type of atom or nucleus passing from the high- to low-energy level is always the same, thus enabling the examiner to determine the quantity and species of atoms present in the specimen and, as we shall see later, where they were located.

RADIO WAVES AND THE ELECTROMAGNETIC SPECTRUM

Nuclear magnetic resonance imaging, however, is somewhat more complex, and at this point it is useful to review where radio waves fit in the entire electromagnetic spectrum. Radio waves are one form of electromagnetic waves. One way of conceptualizing an electromagnetic wave is as a waveform with its electric and magnetic components being perpendicular to each other and perpendicular to the line of the wave's propagation. This is an important consideration to remember in NMR imaging (see Chapter 6) because it is the magnetic component of the electromagnetic wave that interacts with the magnetic field of the tissue protons. The magnetic effects of this interaction will be perpendicular to the line of propagation of the electromagnetic or, in this case, the radio-frequency wave. Thus, the directionality of the radio-frequency pulse used to irradiate tissue in an NMR scanner is critical because in NMR imaging it is very important to change the magnetic vector in the tissue in various specific ways. For now, however, it is sufficient to recall that the magnetic force acts perpendicular to the line of propagation of the radio wave (Fig. 2.1).

Many terms are associated with the waveform characteristic of electromagnetic waves, and in this regard it is important to recall the concept of frequency or hertz (Hz) and its relationship to energy and wavelength. If we were to observe the ocean and see that in a 1-min period 10 waves came ashore, the waves could be said to have a frequency of 10 cycles per minute. Electromagnetic waves are described in a similar fashion. If an electromagnetic wave has one complete cycle in one second, it could be said to be an electromagnetic

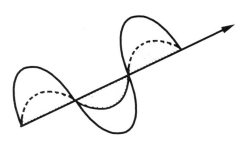

FIG. 2.1. Radio waves are a form of electromagnetic radiation with electric and magnetic components that are perpendicular to the line of propagation indicated by the central vector (*arrow*) in this figure. Thus, the magnetic interaction in NMR scanning is perpendicular to the line of propagation of the radio waves.

wave of 1 Hz. These waves are much faster than ocean waves, and so the frequency or number of hertz observed are by convention usually reported as the number of cycles per second (i.e., number of hertz). The relationship between hertz (frequency), energy, and wavelength for electromagnetic waves is such that waves with increasing hertz have an associated increase in energy but a decrease in wavelength. In reading the rest of this text, it is helpful to remember this direct association between electromagnetic wave energy and increasing hertz and decreasing wavelength.

Within the electromagnetic spectrum, visible light is probably the portion with which we are most familiar. The electromagnetic spectrum is a continuum of waves with both electronic and magnetic properties. In medical diagnosis of the human body, visible light is indeed a very useful portion of the electromagnetic spectrum because many diseases have surface manifestations. However, visible light is not very useful when trying to peer inside the human body. In this regard radiologists have traditionally used the narrow spectrum of fairly high-energy X-rays as a small window (Fig. 2.2) to peer inside

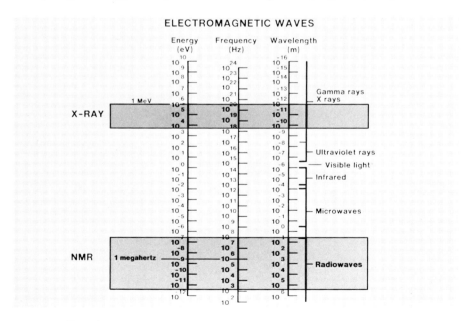

FIG. 2.2. The electromagnetic spectrum is actually a continuum of electromagnetic waves. X-rays, visible light and radio waves are useful in medical diagnosis; however, only X-rays and, more recently, radio waves in conjunction with NMR scanning have been harnessed to act as windows through which to peer inside the body.

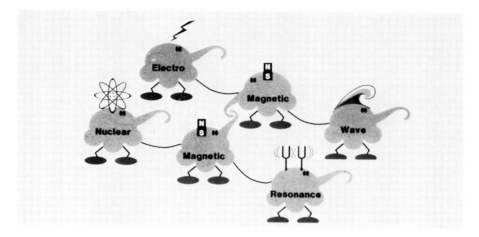

FIG. 2.3. *Zeugmatography* is a term coined by Lauterbur (*zeugma* is a Greek root meaning "yoke" or "to yoke together") indicating that the yoke between electromagnetic waves and NMR is the magnetic interaction between these two forms of energy.

the body and to make the familiar black-and-white X-ray films of bones and other internal organs. Now with the development of NMR imaging, radio waves appear to provide a second small window in the electromagnetic spectrum through which we can look inside the body.

Zeugmatography

Imaging by nuclear magnetic resonance was first described as *zeugmatography* by Lauterbur. This term was intended to imply the joining together (zeugma is the Greek root meaning "a yoke" or "to yoke together") of the magnetic characteristics of nuclear magnetic resonance and electromagnetic waves (Fig. 2.3). The electromagnetic wave emitted from a given nuclear species is characteristic in a static magnetic field, enabling the determination of the nuclear species present. Additionally, a gradient magnetic field can be used to assign the nuclei a position in space within the body.

Chapter 3

Magnets and Magnetic Resonance Concepts

DEFINITIONS

Since magnets have not been used very often in medical imaging in recent times, it might be useful to review briefly some fundamental concepts of magnetism. A magnet is any piece of iron, steel, or originally, a piece of magnetite (loadstone) that has the property of attracting iron or steel, etc. This property may be naturally present or artificially induced by passing an electric current through a coil of wire wrapped around the metal. A magnetic force is the force with which a magnet attracts or repels a piece of iron or steel. Similarly, a magnetic field is the space around the magnet in which its magnetic force is appreciable or measurable.

The gauss (G) is the most common unit of magnetic field strength. One gauss is the measured magnetic field strength at 1 cm from a straight wire carrying a current of 5 amp. Generally speaking, the field strengths used in magnetic resonance imaging are on the order of a few thousand gauss, so the most common magnetic field strength measurements usually encountered will be in the kilogauss range (1000 G). Very high magnetic field strengths are often rated in tesla (T) where 1 T equals 10 kilogauss (KG). The gauss is named after Karl Friedrich Gauss (1777–1855), the German mathematician who made the first absolute measurement of the geomagnetic field of the earth on May 26, 1832. He subsequently devoted much of his scientific life to standardizing and quantifying the measurement of magnetic fields. The tesla was named after Nikola Tesla (1857–1943), an Austrian-born electrician who came to the United States in 1884 and was one of the first to apply the principle of the rotating magnetic field.

15

MAGNETIC FIELDS

Any object that possesses charge and velocity will create a magnetic field. Any positively or negatively charged body moving linearly has a magnetic field that is perpendicular to it, the so-called linear magnetic moment. However, a charged body that is spinning will produce an angular magnetic moment with a magnetic vector perpendicular to the rotational axis (Fig. 3.1).

We are all probably more familiar with the generation of these angular magnetic moments than we realize. For example, the north and south magnetic poles of the earth are produced by similar circumstances. The spinning of the earth creates an angular magnetic moment that results in the earth's magnetic field, and in the same sense, a magnetic field is produced by charged nuclear particles spinning within body tissues. This principle is extremely important in magnetic resonance imaging. An equally important comparison with the earth's magnetic field is the fact that its magnetic field strength is not uniform but rather weaker at the equator (approximately 0.3 G) than it is at the north pole (approximately 0.7 G). Thus, there is a gradient in the earth's magnetic field, and by measuring it we could

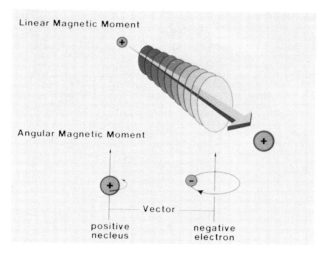

FIG. 3.1. Moving charged particles create a magnetic field called a magnetic moment. Charge particles moving in a linear fashion create a circular magnetic field perpendicular to the line of movement, whereas charged particles which are spinning create an angular magnetic moment whose vector is perpendicular to the rotation of the small charged particle.

determine whether we were at the equator or at the pole or anywhere in between (Fig. 3.2). In a similar manner, gradient magnetic fields are used in NMR imaging to determine spatial localization within tissues.

In this book we are primarily concerned with the atomic nucleus in tissue as the component to be exploited in imaging, and we will use the earth as an analogy for the atomic nucleus in order to help explain the imaging process. To make this transition, we will compare the angular magnetic moment of the earth with the angular magnetic moment of the nucleus—in this case, the hydrogen nucleus or proton ^1H in tissue is the most useful. Both the earth and the ^1H nucleus spin on an axis. This spinning creates a magnetic field around these bodies, and the net sum of the magnetic field is perpendicular to the axis rotation. This magnetic field can be represented as a dipole magnet or as a magnetic vector indicating direction and magnitude representing the sum of the entire field strength (Fig. 3.3). This, henceforth, is the way the magnetic dipole of spinning nuclei will be represented in this book.

There are many atomic nuclear species that possess net charge and spin, and therefore possess a small magnetic moment. However, some nuclei do not have net spin and magnetic moment.

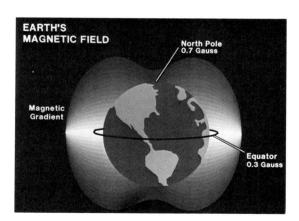

FIG. 3.2. The magnetic field of the earth is one example of angular magnetic moment produced by the rotation of the earth on its axis. The magnetic field is somewhat stronger at the north and south poles than it is at the equator, and by knowing this relationship and the field strength at any given point, one could locate his or her latitude on the earth's surface.

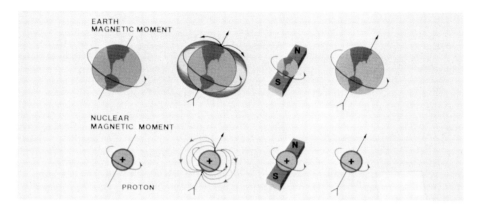

FIG. 3.3. In NMR imaging the hydrogen nucleus, which is composed of a single proton, and its magnetic field can be compared with the magnetic field of the earth. Both the earth and proton nucleus spin on an axis. This rotation generates a magnetic field whose vector is perpendicular to the angle of rotation and causes it to function as if it were a magnet with a north and south pole. This magnetic dipole, as it is called, is usually represented by a vector indicating the strength and direction of the net magnetic fields.

THE NATURE OF SPINNING PARTICLES

The magnitude of angular magnetic moment depends on both the angular momentum (mass × velocity) and charge. Total angular momentum for electrons depends on both their spin and their orbital angular momentum. The majority of nuclei also possess spin although the angular momentum concerned varies from nucleus to nucleus. The simplest nucleus is that of the hydrogen atom, which consists of one particle only, the proton. The proton also has a spin of one-half, designated as S. Another particle that is a constituent of all other nuclei is the neutron; this has a unit mass equal to that of the proton but no charge and again a spin of one-half. Thus, if a particular nucleus is composed of P (protons) and N (neutrons), its total mass is P + N and its total charge is + P, and its total spin will be a vector combination of P + N spins, each of magnitude one-half. The atomic mass is usually specified for each nucleus by writing it as a prefix to the nuclear symbol, i.e., ^{12}C, which indicates that the nucleus of a carbon has a mass of 12. Since the atomic charge is 6 for this nucleus, we know immediately that the nucleus must have 6 protons and 6 neutrons to make up a mass of 12. The nucleus ^{13}C (an isotope of carbon) has 6 protons and 7 neutrons. In NMR imaging it is the unpaired nuclear particles that confer the magnetic moment on the nucleus. Thus, ^{12}C, having an equal number of protons and neutrons, cannot be magnetized, whereas the isotope ^{13}C is magnetized and can be used in a special type of NMR imaging called chemical shift imaging (see Chapter 8).

Each nuclear species, being composed of a different number of protons and neutrons, will have its own total spin value, and depending on these values, plus the nuclear charge, there may be a strong or absent nuclear magnetic moment.

Without going into more detail, the following generalizations can be made:

1. Nuclei with both P and N even have zero spin (i.e., ^{4}He, ^{12}C, ^{16}O, etc.)
2. Nuclei with both P and N odd (has charge odd, but mass [P + N] even) have integral spin (i.e., ^{2}H, ^{14}N [spin equal 1] ^{10}B [spin equal 3], etc.)
3. Nuclei with odd nuclear mass have one-half integral spins (i.e., ^{1}N, ^{15}N, [spin = 1/2], ^{17}O [spin = 5/2], etc.)

In general, a charged particle spinning about an axis constitutes a circular electric current that in turn produces a magnetic dipole. In other words, the spinning charged particle behaves as a tiny bar magnet placed along the spin axis.

Chapter 4

Nuclear Magnetic Resonance Principles

NET MAGNETIZATION

Net magnetization (M) at rest is zero. In body tissues, or any specimen for that matter, before the application of a magnetic field, the magnetic moments of the nuclei making up the tissue are randomly aligned, as shown in Fig. 4.1, and have zero net magnetization (M = 0). When an external fixed magnetic field is applied, after an interval, the individual magnetic moments align parallel or antiparallel with the applied net magnetic field, B. There is a slight preponderance of nuclei aligned parallel with the magnetic field, and this gives the tissue a net magnetization (M) (Fig. 4.2). As an example for ^1H, which has a large magnetic moment in a field of 14 kilogauss (KG), the fractional excess of parallel protons is only about 1×10^{-5} at room temperature. Nevertheless, as small as this slight excess is, it accounts for the small macroscopic net magnetic moment directed parallel with the external magnetic field, and it is this differential that accounts for the nuclear magnetic resonance signal on which the imaging is based.

Another important difference between the parallel and antiparallel protons is that the antiparallel protons are at a slightly higher energy level than the parallel protons. One way to conceptualize this difference in energy states is to consider the different levels of energy expended by two swimmers both tied to ropes and attempting to swim toward each other with one swimming downstream (with the static magnetic field) and the other expending more energy while swimming upstream (against the static magnetic field).

In NMR imaging the energy differential between the parallel and antiparallel protons is directly proportional to external field strength (Fig. 4.3). The energy differential (ΔE) is given by the equation $\Delta E = [\gamma h/2\pi] B$ where γ is the magnetogyric ratio and B is the external

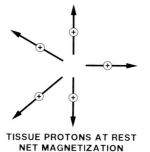

TISSUE PROTONS AT REST
NET MAGNETIZATION
(M = O)

FIG. 4.1. In the absence of an external magnetic field, the magnetic dipoles or vectors of the protons in the tissue align randomly so that there is no net tissue magnetization.

field strength. At this point the important thing to note about these different energy levels is that the energy differential approximates the thermal energy exchanged between colliding molecules and thus is quite small, i.e., on the order of a few millicalories. At any given field strength, the two energy levels resonate. The energy exchange is at a very specific level, and the higher the magnetic field strength is, the greater the difference between the energies of the parallel and antiparallel protons.

MAGNETIC WOBBLE

So far we have represented the magnetic moment of the ensemble of protons in tissue as being in stable alignment with the external static magnetic field. In actuality each one of these magnetic moments wobbles or rotates around the alignment of the static magnetic field in a process that is called *precession*. By way of analogy, the interaction between the proton angular magnetic moment and the external magnetic field, and the spinning mass of a top and the earth's gravitation field are similar interactions, with the exception that the competing forces acting on a wobbling top are the earth's static grav-

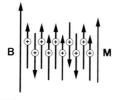

TISSUE PROTONS IN EXTERNAL
MAGNETIC FIELD (B)
WITH NET MAGNETIZATION (M)

FIG. 4.2. Protons in an external magnetic field (B) align either parallel or antiparallel with the external field and the nature of this alignment is such that a small number are aligned parallel with the external field which in turn confers a net magnetization of the sample or tissue (M).

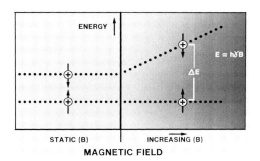

FIG. 4.3. Protons that are parallel with the static magnetic field (B) are at a slightly lower energy level than those aligned antiparallel with the static magnetic field. The energy difference between these two states is directly related to the strength of the external magnetic field such that the energy difference increases with increasing field strength.

itational field trying to push the top down versus the top's angular momentum attempting to keep the top upright (Fig. 4.4). Thus, in a friction-free system, a top spinning on a flat surface possesses a resonant precession or wobble about the direction of the local gravitational field. In a similar manner, a spinning nucleus also precesses or wobbles about an applied magnetic field with a resonant angular frequency, determined by a constant (the magnetogyric ratio, γ) and the strength of the magnetic field B. Each nuclear species possesses a characteristic value for γ but ω and B are related by the equation $\omega = \gamma B$. The important relationship in this equation is that the angular frequency for any nuclear species is characteristic and directly

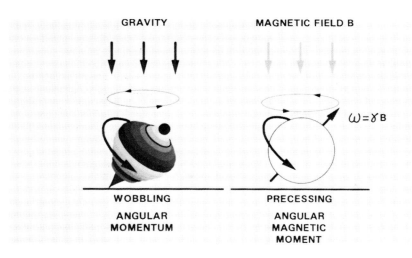

FIG. 4.4. Protons in an external magnetic field do not remain in one position; they wobble or precess around the applied force of the external magnetic field in the same way that a top wobbles in a gravitational field. The frequency (ω) at which the proton precesses is directly related to the strength, B, of the external magnetic field ($\omega = \gamma B$). (γ = magnetogyric ratio.)

proportional to the static magnetic field. Thus, there is an interrelationship between ω and E, such that both resonant frequency (ω) and proton energy (E) are directly proportional to the magnetic field: E = h γB; ω = γB; γ = Magnetogyric ratio; h = Planck's constant; and B = Magnetic field.

Chapter 5

Nuclear Magnetic Resonance and Electromagnetic Waves

RESONANCE

All of us are probably more familiar with the concepts of resonance than we are aware. In the experiment from high school science using two tuning forks, both of which are tuned to the note C, one tuning fork is struck and placed next to the other and the second tuning fork begins to vibrate and emit the note C. This second tone will continue even if the first tuning fork is removed. The first tuning fork is said to have made the second tuning fork resonate and emit the same tone (Fig. 5.1). To explore this concept slightly further, if we now take the C tuning fork and place it in a room in which there are several tuning forks that have different tones (resonant frequencies), for example, the notes F, A, C, and E, indicated in Fig. 5.2, and again strike the C tuning fork, a peculiar phenomenon occurs. Even though they are all tuning forks, only the tuning fork that emits the letter C will begin to vibrate (resonate). All of the other tuning forks seem to ignore the presence of the vibrating C tuning fork in the room.

You will recall from Chapter 2 on electromagnetic waves that frequency and energy are directly related. What is occurring in this

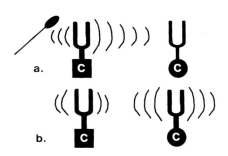

FIG. 5.1. The principle of resonance is probably most easily illustrated with tuning forks. If a tuning fork of a given tone C is struck with a mallet and placed in proximity to another tuning fork of the same tone, the second tuning fork will begin to vibrate and similarly emit the tone C. The seconding tuning fork can be said to have been made to resonate (produce the tone C) by absorbing the energy of the first tuning fork. This resonance of the tone C will persist even if the first tuning fork is removed.

"tuning fork example" is that energy is imparted to the C tuning fork as we strike it with the mallet. This energy then is transformed into sonic waves with a certain *frequency* or number of hertz per second, which we hear as the *tone* or the note C, and the note's *amplitude* we hear as the *loudness* of the tone C. This energy then is transmitted across the room to all the tuning forks present, but only the C tuning fork is able to absorb that specific energy, and that energy causes the arms to vibrate, subsequently reemitting (resonating) the appropriate frequency, the tone C.

Throughout this book, many of the principles of magnetic resonance will be explained in terms of analogies with sonic waves. It is important to remember, however, that sonic waves are not electromagnetic waves. But they do have certain characteristics analogous to electromagnetic waves like wavelength, frequency, and energy or amplitude.

In NMR imaging, electromagnetic waves can exist as single monochromatic frequencies and two waves with the same amplitude can

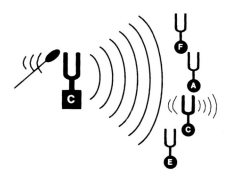

FIG. 5.2. If several tuning forks are placed in proximity to a tuning fork which has been struck with a mallet, only the tuning fork with the same tone (resonant frequency) will absorb the specific or characteristic energy and begin to resonate. The other tuning forks are not capable of absorbing the energy from an unmatched tone. In other words the energy exchange must occur at a very specific or characteristic level or tone.

be determined from each other if they have different frequencies (Fig. 5.3). The same wave can be represented in one of two ways: either as a wave of given amplitude and duration (time domain) or as a frequency distribution of waves (frequency domain) (Fig. 5.4). In addition, many waves of different frequencies and amplitudes can be superimposed on each other and represented as one wave with frequency and amplitude modulation (see Fig. 5.4). In NMR imaging, these characteristics of frequency and amplitude or energy are used in making images of the body by separating a complex series of radio-frequency (RF) signals emitted from the nuclei into their components of frequency and amplitude. The frequency is used to locate a particular position of the nucleus within the body, and the amplitude is used to determine the number of nuclei present at that location. The tuning fork example illustrates an important principle in magnetic resonance such that for any given ensemble of different tuning forks, only a very specific or characteristic energy (tone) can be absorbed by any one of them. But this characteristic energy or tone can be exchanged between any tuning forks that have the same tone. Those that are not vibrating can be said to be at rest or at a lower energy state than those that have been excited or induced to vibrate either by being struck directly or by absorbing energy from another vibrating tuning fork. This essentially illustrates the principle in quantum mechanics in which particles, such as proton nuclei, achieve only very specific energy states. The energy required to convert them

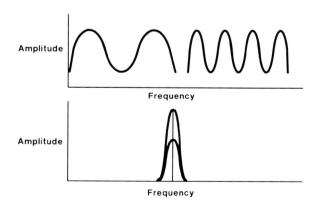

FIG. 5.3. In NMR imaging the radio-frequency waves in the NMR signal can have the same amplitude but different frequencies (*top graph*) or two waves can have the same frequency but different amplitudes, and they can potentially be separated from each other on this basis.

FIG. 5.4. Radio-frequency (RF) electromagnetic waves in the NMR signal are usually modulated or superimposed on each other resulting in complex amplitudes and frequencies, as illustrated in the time domain of A + B *(bottom graph)*. Fortunately, using a complex mathematical digital computer program called the *fast Fourier transform,* these complex amplitude waveforms in the time domain can be converted to

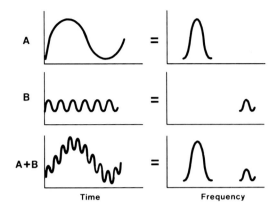

separable amplitude waveforms in the frequency domain, and this frequency resolution can be used to locate the part of the body from which the radiofrequency signal was sent.

from one to the other must be exactly at that level in order to achieve the change in energy state, and higher energies or lower energies will not produce the change. In other words, the absorbed and emitted energy in atomic particles is characteristic or very specific for that atom or nucleus, just as the tone C is characteristic or very specific for the C tuning fork in the above example.

Magnetic resonance, however, implies an interaction between a magnet and a magnetic field rather than a physical interaction of sonic waves. For most of us, the most familiar interaction of a magnet with a magnetic field is the interaction of a compass needle (permanent bar magnet mounted on a needle fulcrum) and the magnetic field of the earth. At rest the compass needle is aligned with the earth's magnetic field pointing north. If the compass needle is deflected with your finger, it will swing back toward its resting position, overshoot, and oscillate back and forth at some frequency, eventually coming to rest again pointing north. This frequency of oscillation is called the *natural frequency,* and for any given point in the magnetic field of the earth and any given compass needle, the frequency is characteristic. Because of this relationship between a compass needle's natural frequency and the magnetic field of the earth, we could determine with this system our latitude on the earth or spatial location. If our compass had a natural frequency of 1 Hz at the equator with 0.3 G field strength and if we moved to a new position in which the natural frequency was 2 Hz, we would know we were at a latitude that was near the north pole corresponding to a magnetic field strength twice that of the equator, or 0.6 G magnetic field strength. We would also know whether we were north or south of the equator by determining whether we were traveling toward or away from the north pointing compass in getting to the new position (Fig. 5.5). In other words, using the frequency of the compass, we can determine (spatially encode) our latitudinal position. In NMR imaging, the magnet is, of course, not a compass needle but the magnetic moment of an atomic nucleus, usually hydrogen. The magnetic field in NMR is a very strong magnetic field, approximately 4,000 to 40,000 times that of the earth or greater, induced by the surrounding magnet of the NMR imaging system.

EXCITATION

Carrying these concepts further and extending them to NMR sample or *in vitro* tissue experiments, the protons or nuclei are generally in an unaligned (Fig. 4.1) state and with zero magnetization, as discussed in Chapter 4. However, when the tissue is placed in an external static magnetic field, the protons align with the external magnetic field. If, as in Fig. 5.6, some are receptive and able to resonate when a specific frequency signal is applied to the tissue, in this case, "hello," they will be excited to a higher energy state antiparallel to the static magnetic field, after the absorption of their characteristic frequency ("hello"). Some time later, however, they will flip back to the parallel lower energy level with simultaneous emission of the frequency that caused them to flip over in the first

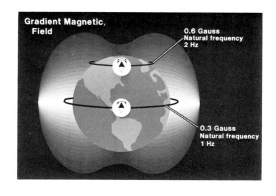

FIG. 5.5. A compass needle at the equator experiencing a magnetic field of approximately 0.3 G will oscillate at its natural frequency after it is deflected. This natural frequency of oscillation is influenced by the magnetic field in which the compass is placed such that doubling the magnetic field will double the natural frequency of oscillation. In this way, if we were given a natural frequency of 1 Hz at the equator and placed in a new position on the earth in which the natural frequency of oscillation was observed to have increased to 2 Hz, we could correctly locate our position at that latitude corresponding to exactly twice the magnetic field of the equator or 0.6 G.

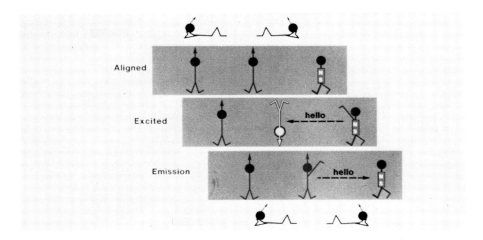

FIG. 5.6. Protons in the absence of an external magnetic field are randomly aligned with no net tissue magnetization; however, when placed in the presence of an external magnetic field, they become aligned with the field and can be stimulated (excited) to change alignment by the absorption of a specific frequency signal—in this case, "hello." The protons after some period of time then lose the energy (hello) and become realigned in their initial orientation (emission). Removal of the external magnetic field will again cause random alignment of the protons and zero net magnetization.

place ("hello"). The removal of the magnetic field will again cause a random alignment of the protons in the tissue and zero net magnetization. This principle is called *resonance* and indicates the process by which nuclei absorb energy (RF energy) when the transmitted radio frequency matches the resonant frequency of the nuclei.

RESONANCE IN NUCLEAR MAGNETIC RESONANCE

Similarly, when imaging the human body, the spinning protons in an organ align either parallel or antiparallel with an externally imposed magnetic field. The protons pointing in the parallel direction are at a slightly lower energy level than those pointing in the antiparallel direction, as previously illustrated in Figure 4.3. The energy difference $\Delta E = hB\gamma$ is on the order of magnitude of the thermal energy generated in random collisions of the protons (molecules) with their environments (approximately 6 millicalories). Thus, protons in the magnetic field tend to alternate back and forth between the parallel and antiparallel states absorbing and/or emitting energy as they collide with their surrounding environment. A short time after the application of the static magnetic field, the number of protons pointing in the parallel direction slightly outnumber those pointing in antiparallel direction and the sample is said to be magnetized (M). The difference is small and on the order of 1 nucleus/10^6 nuclei.

In a static magnetic field, similar to those used in clinical imaging with magnetic resonance (approximately 2 KG), the energy required to stimulate or excite a low-energy parallel proton to a higher energy antiparallel proton is the energy of electromagnetic waves in the RF (short wave) scale (approximately 4 MHz [mega Hertz]) or 10^{-8} eV [electron volts] (see Fig. 2.2). Thus, if in a static field, RF waves of the right frequency are passed through the sample, some of the parallel protons will absorb energy and be stimulated or excited to a higher energy in the antiparallel direction. At some time later, the exact RF frequency absorbed will be emitted as electromagnetic energy of the same frequency as the RF source. The protons continue to absorb-emit, absorb-emit (i.e., to resonate), as long as the radio waves have the correct resonant frequency. In general, resonance is a relationship between matching frequencies such that the exchange of energy is at discrete levels, and the RF that is emitted by the resonating protons is the signal that eventually generates the NMR image in medical imaging.

Actually, the exact amount of energy required to flip a proton from the parallel to the antiparallel orientation (and thus a higher energy state) is directly related to the magnetic field strength; stronger fields require more energy (see Fig. 4.3). This greater energy is furnished by higher frequency radio waves (since the energy of any electromagnetic irradiation is in direct proportion to its frequency). Therefore, the frequency required to excite a proton is a direct function of the imposed magnetic field. A stronger field will require higher frequency radiation. For a magnetic field strength of 3.5 KG, the appropriate radio wave has a frequency of 15 MHz and wavelength of 20 m.

Nuclear Magnetic Resonance: Terms Reviewed

Thus, we now have the full dimension of the terminology of nuclear magnetic resonance in mind; *nuclear* because the magnetic moment used in this technique is provided by spinning charged nuclear particles such as the proton in hydrogen; *magnetic,* because the tissue sample is magnetized in an external static magnetic field due to the slight preponderance of parallel to antiparallel protons in the tissue;

and *resonance* because the RF and precessional frequency are identical. The exchange of energy (RF waves) between the low- and high-energy protons in the sample is an exchange of energy at discrete, specific, characteristic levels. The RF of the resonating protons is the signal from which the NMR image is eventually generated.

THE NUCLEAR MAGNETIC RESONANCE SIGNAL

Before moving forward to a discussion of the techniques used in imaging with magnetic resonance, let us consider in a little more detail the nature of the magnetic resonance signal itself. If we review another high school physics experiment, in which a bar magnet is moved perpendicular to a coil with a voltmeter on it, we see that a current is induced. Similarly, if we represent the bar magnet as a vector with direction and magnitude, as that magnetic vector sweeps past a metal coil, a current will be induced, which can be measured (see Fig. 5.11). Although in actual practice, magnetic resonance imaging is performed using the emitted RF signal, there is a relationship between the emitted RF signal and a change in the vector of the net magnetization of the tissue, and the two can be thought of somewhat interchangeably. For the purposes of explanation, it is sometimes easier to think in terms of a voltage induced in a coil rather than the RF signal recorded in a receiver coil. But the reader should bear in mind that in practice, it is the RF signal that is actually being measured. Also note that the FIO signal on the osciliscope is the beats of the RF signal and not the RF frequency itself.

Principles

As we are ultimately working toward an explanation of magnetic resonance imaging and as we will be discussing the representation of various internal organs in three dimensions, we should begin to think of the following discussions in terms of three-dimensional space. In representing this, it is easiest to represent body tissues in terms of three intersecting perpendicular planes. To avoid having to draw the perpendicular planes in each figure, however, the three planes will be indicated by three intersecting x, y, and z axes with the z axis indicating the alignment of the static external magnetic field (Fig. 5.7). In addition, when we are using the principles of classical Newtonian electromagnetic theory, vectors (arrows) are used extensively to represent the direction and magnitude of net tissue magnetization.

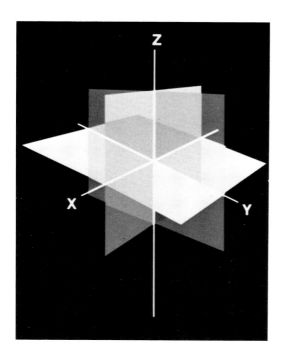

FIG. 5.7. In NMR imaging the magnetic fields of the scanners are generally oriented in three intersecting perpendicular planes. These three planes can be represented as x, y, and z axes, and magnetic vectors lying along these axes can be represented as arrows with direction and magnitude. For simplicity throughout the remainder of the text, only the axes will be depicted. However, the reader should recall that these axes are representing three intersecting planes.

Proton Density T_1 and T_2 Relaxation

To review the preceding discussion, a tissue at rest has zero net magnetization (M). However, in a static external magnetic field, the protons (all magnetic nuclei, in fact) align parallel or antiparallel to the static magnetic field, and since there is a slight excess of parallel protons ($1/10^6$), the tissue has a slight magnetization. We can represent this net magnetization as M, and since this is aligned along the static magnetic field axis, we can indicate it as being M_z (Fig. 5.8). One way to change the direction of net magnetization would be to simply apply another magnetic field to the tissue, say with a bar magnet (Fig. 5.9). If applied appropriately along the y axis, this would cause net tissue magnetization to shift slightly from the z axis with some resultant angle α to the x,y plane.

Another way to accomplish the same end result would be to use a RF (electromagnetic) pulse at the resonant frequency of the protons in the tissue. As we discussed in Chapter 4, in a manner similar to a spinning top, a proton will precess about the vertical axis of an external magnetic field. If we wish to change the axis of these protons,

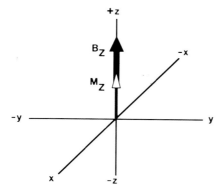

FIG. 5.8. The magnitude and direction of the external magnetic field is represented by a vector (B_z) as is the magnitude and direction of net tissue magnetization (M_z). In this figure both the external magnetic field and net tissue magnetization are oriented along the z axis, and in many NMR scanners this axis is parallel with the long axis of the body and the long axis of the scanner.

the RF wave form is particularly well suited to applying a constant torque or force. Because the proton is precessing in the main field, the second field needs to oscillate at the precessional frequency in order to apply a constant force. This oscillating magnetic field re-

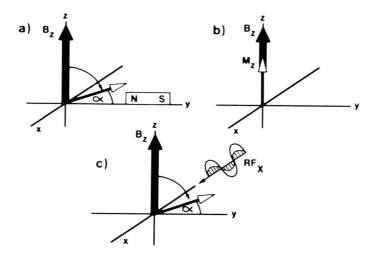

FIG. 5.9. In NMR imaging it is important to attempt to change the axis of net tissue magnetization (M_z). One way of approaching this change would be simply to place a bar magnet in the desired direction, in this case, along the y axis (a), resulting in a deflection of the net tissue magnetization to a new angle. Moving the bar magnets around in such a fashion would be very difficult within an NMR scanner, and in practice the magnetic force is applied using an electromagnetic wave in the radio-frequency range (RF pulse). Recalling from Chapter 2 that the magnetic force acts perpendicular to the line of propagation of the RF wave in order to rotate M_z to the new angle, the pulse should be applied along the x axis, i.e., RF_x.

quired is ideally provided by the waveform of an electromagnetic wave in the RF range, i.e., a radio wave. This magnetic torque when applied to the proton causes a rotation about the horizontal axis (Fig. 5.10). As before, the specific resonant frequency is determined by the local value of the magnetic field. During each precessional cycle, the torque due to the radio wave causes the proton axis to rotate slowly (i.e., be deflected) until it eventually lies along the y axis, 90° from where it started. The amount of RF energy needed to do this is called a 90° pulse (Fig. 5.10). In addition, the net magnetic moment or magnetization M now precesses with the same characteristic frequency ω because the individual magnetic moments causing this shift in NMR are all in phase with the applied radio waves. A precessing magnetic vector induces an NMR signal (Hz) or voltage in a receiver coil if it is precessing perpendicular to it the same way a moving bar magnet produces a voltage in a wire coil (Fig. 5.11). When using a description based on classical or Newtonian physics, we should really speak of large groups or ensembles of protons rather than just one. The formula relating these events is ω = γB, where γ is the

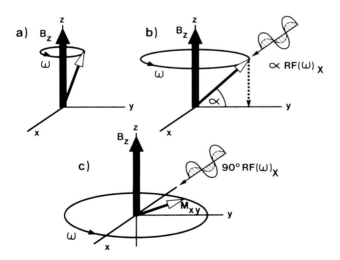

FIG. 5.10. Net tissue magnetization (M_z) actually precesses about the external magnetic field (B_z) and the waveform of the RF pulse is ideal to apply a constant torque to this rotating vector. The amount of rotation is related to the duration and amplitude of the applied RF pulse. An RF pulse of sufficient duration and power to rotate M_z through 90° is referred to as the 90° RF (ω_x) pulse, with ω indicating that the RF pulse needs to be applied at the resonant frequency of the precessing magnetic moment M_z.

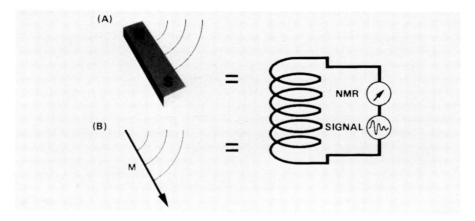

FIG. 5.11. Following the RF pulse the transverse magnetization M_{xy} precesses around the axis of the external field, inducing an a.c. signal in the receiver coil in the same way a bar magnet moved in the same plane would induce a signal. Since precession occurs at the Larmor frequency, the voltage induced in the coil is of the same frequency (ω), however the signal is viewed as beats on the CRT.

magnetogyric ratio and B again is the magnetic field. The ω is the resonant angular frequency. It should be remembered that cyclical frequency f is less than the angular frequency: $f = \omega/2\pi$. ω is the Larmor or characteristic resonant angular frequency.

As might be anticipated, the angle of deflection or rotation of tissue net magnetization (α) depends primarily on the product of the amplitude and length of the applied RF pulse. It is possible to shift the net magnetization vector (M) to any desired angle (α) of deflection by applying the resonant frequency pulse (αRF) for the appropriate amount of time. The M can, in fact, be completely inverted (Fig. 5.12), and the appropriate pulse is called 180° RF_x pulse, i.e., 180° RF_x is an RF pulse applied along the x axis to achieve a 180° shift around the x axis.

When the RF pulse is turned off, however, the net tissue magnetization begins to swing back toward the positive z axis inducing an NMR signal in the appropriately placed receiver coil that must be perpendicular to the moving magnetic vector (Fig. 5.13).

The size or magnitude of the NMR signal received by the coil is proportional to the number of proton nuclei in the tissue. In addition, the time required after the 180° RF_x pulse for the net tissue magnetization to return from negative (M_{-z}) to positive (M_{+z}) is called the

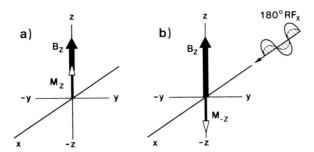

FIG. 5.12. In practical terms M_z can be rotated through any desired degree of rotation but commonly the two pulse sequences used are 180° RF_x, resulting in an inversion M_z to M_{-z}, and a 90° RF_x.

relaxation time and is referred to in NMR terminology as T_1, or the T_1 relaxation time.

T_1 RELAXATION TIME

Proton density, as we have reviewed above, is a very important aspect of the NMR signal and relates much information regarding the type of substance or tissue being evaluated. The total NMR signal has much more information in it than just the number and type of nuclei reflected in the amplitude of the signal. One can also charac-

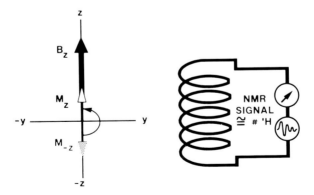

FIG. 5.13. After inversion M_{-z} returns to M_z after an appropriate time interval. During this process, the magnetic vector changes and the protons emit the NMR signal (RF signal), which can be detected by a receiver coil, and the signal, viewed as beats rather than the RF frequency, is generally proportional to the number of proton nuclei present in the sample.

terize a given substance or tissue by the way the nuclei relax. Relaxation in NMR refers to the time required for the net tissue magnetization vectors to come to or return to equilibrium conditions in a static external magnetic field.

T_1 relaxation can be illustrated by referring back to the compass analogy (see Fig. 5.5). We noted that a compass needle in the earth's magnetic field would oscillate at a frequency that was characteristic for that needle at a specific point in the earth's magnetic field. At this point we should also consider the duration of oscillation over time. If we take a compass in the earth's magnetic field and place it within a wire coil connected to a voltage source and subsequently deflect the needle, a damped signal will be recorded in the coil perpendicular to the angle of oscillation of the compass needle, and the duration of this decay from beginning to end will have a certain finite time, which we can refer to as the relaxation time of the compass needle, or the time required after stimulation for the compass needle to return to equilibrium conditions. Conceptually, T_1 relaxation times in NMR are a very similar phenomenon. For purposes of illustration, we can return to the vector analysis originally presented in Fig. 5.9 and extend it here in Fig. 5.14.

Net tissue magnetization (M_z) is at equilibrium with the external magnetic field B_z. However, if we induce net tissue magnetization to become inverted (M_{-z}) with a bar magnet or, in the case of NMR, with a RF pulse, net tissue magnetization will slowly return to its resting position (M_z). M at any time after M_z inversion to M_{-z} can be represented as either a negative or positive vector along the z axis,

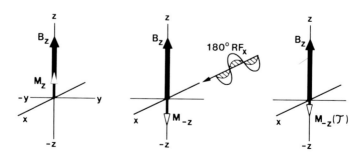

FIG. 5.14. If net tissue magnetization (M_z) is inverted with a 180° RF_x pulse, net tissue magnetization will slowly return from the M_{-z} position to its original M_z position. This process is called *relaxation* and begins as soon as the 180° RF_x pulse is terminated, as illustrated by the shorter M_{-z} vector that occurs at some time τ after cessation of the 180° RF pulse.

and a general case can be illustrated as $M_{-z}(\tau)$, with τ being some time interval after the initial inversion stimulation (Fig. 5.14).

In practice, changes in net tissue magnetization along the z axis cannot be measured because of the configuration of the NMR scanners. Therefore, purely as a practical technique in measuring T_1, M_z is deflected toward the coil by following the 180° RF pulse with a 90° RF pulse (Fig. 5.15). This process is repeated for several different time intervals (τ) following the initial M_z inversion and the measurement of the magnitude of M_{-z}. After several measurements, the exact time of T_1 can be determined, as illustrated in Fig. 5.16. Because this relaxation occurs along the z axis or is parallel to or longitudinal with the static magnetic field, this form of T_1 relaxation is sometimes referred to as *longitudinal relaxation*.

T_2 RELAXATION TIME

Thus, we have now two methods within the NMR signal to describe a given tissue or sample. One is the density of the nuclei (proton nuclei within that sample as determined by the amplitude of the NMR signal), and the second is the time it takes the net magnetization of the tissue or sample to return to its equilibrium position along the z axis after some magnetic deflection.

The third parameter is T_2. Everyone has had the experience of throwing a pebble in a small pond and watching the wave spread out in a circular fashion until it has traversed the entire surface of the pond. The time is dependent on the size of the pond, and if the pond is not too large, the wave is visible throughout its course over the

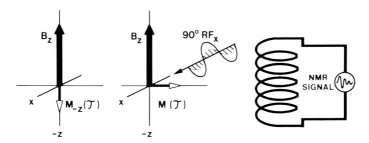

FIG. 5.15. Because of the way most NMR imaging systems are constructed, changes of M_z along the z axis cannot be directly measured. Therefore, in this type of imaging, which is referred to as *inversion recovery*, a 90° RF_x pulse is applied at variable intervals after the 180° RF_x is applied so that the signal can be measured from the RF transmitter-receiver coil.

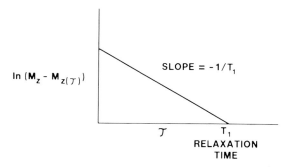

FIG. 5.16. By obtaining several measurements at variable intervals τ after the 180° RF$_x$ pulse, the time required for M$_{-z}$ to return to M$_{+z}$ can be measured. This time interval is referred to as the T$_1$ relaxation time, and because it occurs along the z axis, in alignment with the external magnetic field, it is therefore sometimes called the *longitudinal relaxation time.* The relaxation time is the time constant 1/T$_1$. Complete relaxation occurs approximately 3 to 4 × T$_1$.

surface. If we take a handful of pebbles, however, and throw them into the pond, the effect of the waveforms on the surface is quite different. Although each wave initially starts out as did the single wave from the single pebble, the wave fronts very quickly encounter each other leaving no discernable single wave and the surface again "appears" smooth as if the waves have vanished. In fact , this is not true, the waves are still traversing the surface but the superimposition of crests and troughs tends to cancel each other out. The smoothing of the surface by wave interference is similar to what happens in T$_2$ relaxation.

An analogy to sonic waves is apt here. If we take, for example, a room full of tuning forks all tuned to the tone C and strike each one of them individually and simultaneously, we would have a very loud C tone with loudness proportional to the number of tuning forks in the room (Fig. 5.17). If instead we take a soldering iron and apply variable amounts of solder to each one of the tuning forks so that each resonant tone is just slightly different than the tone C and again strike all of the tuning forks simultaneously, we would initially hear again a very loud C tone. This time, however, the sound would quickly fade away and we would hear no sound at all. If we inspect the tuning forks, they would appear to be still vibrating even though no tone would be audible. If one of the tuning forks is picked up and taken out of the room as we move into the hallway, we again would hear the tone emanating from the tuning fork (Fig. 5.18). Returning

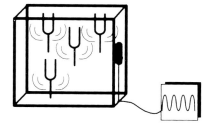

FIG. 5.17. Tuning forks tuned to the same tone enclosed in a room, if struck, will emit a loud tone that can be detected by a microphone.

to the room, we again would note that the tone is quickly damped and shortly thereafter inaudible.

The reason for this phenomenon is similar to the disruption of the visual pattern of the waves on the surface of the pond. Because each of the tuning forks was tuned slightly differently due to the applied solder, the sonic waves did not reinforce each other but rather dephased very quickly and resulted in mutual cancellation of their tones even though all were continuing to vibrate (Fig. 5.18).

In NMR the explanation of T_2 relaxation time has comparisons with both of these analogies, although neither is exactly transferable because the cancellation phenomenon in T_2 relaxation time is a cancellation of the individual magnetic moments of the precessing protons rather than a waveform interference.

The classical Newtonian electromagnetic model follows: In a body before application of a magnetic field, the magnetic moments of the nuclei making up the tissue are randomly aligned as previously discussed. When a magnetic field is applied, individual magnetic moments attempt to align with the direction of the applied magnetic field B_z but precess around it. As these magnetic moments are randomly

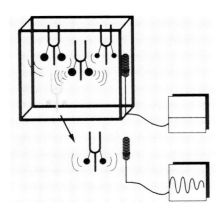

FIG. 5.18. If tuning forks, which were originally tuned to the same tone, have variable small weights attached to their arms, and then are induced to vibrate, a microphone enclosed within the room will detect no tone at all because of the phase interference among the tuning forks produced by the small weights. If one of the tuning forks is removed from the room, however, a tone will be recorded because the dampening effect of wave interference has been removed. In NMR scanning T_2 relaxation involves a similar kind of cancellation among proton magnetic moments that rapidly dephase.

oriented with respect to one another, the components in the xy plane cancel one another out and $M_{xy} = 0$ while the M_z components along the direction of the applied magnetic field do not cancel each other and produce a net magnetic moment M_z (Fig. 5.19).

If the material or tissue is now irradiated with a radio wave at resonant frequency ω, with the precessing nuclei (rotating magnetic field RF_x), two things occur simultaneously:

1. The net tissue magnetization (M_z) will be rotated away from the z axis, as shown in Fig. 5.19. The angle of rotation α depends primarily on the duration of the applied RF pulse (α = Kt_p, where t_p is the pulse length in seconds and K is a constant).

2. The individual magnetic moments are brought into the same phase (coherence) with the applied RF pulse and the net magnetic moment (M) now precesses with the same characteristic frequency ω in the xy plane.

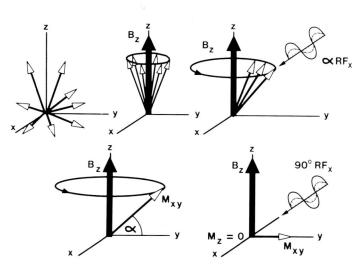

FIG. 5.19. The magnetic moments of the randomly aligned protons precess about the z axis in the presence of an external magnetic field (B_z). This orientation results in a net tissue magnetization along the z axis (M_z), but because they are randomly aligned with respect to the xy axes, no magnetic moment is recorded in the xy plane. However, when an RF pulse is applied, two things occur simultaneously. First, the net tissue magnetization begins to rotate about the x axis; second, the RF pulse causes the randomly aligned proton magnetic moments to become coherent with respect to the xy plane, and they tend to precess together. If the RF pulse applied is appropriate for a 90° rotation (90° RF_x), then the magnetic moments will be coherently aligned in the xy plane resulting in a magnetic moment in the xy plane, (M_{xy}) but no net tissue magnetization will be recorded on the z axis ($M_z = 0$). Note: In the static reference frame M_z spirals down to the xy plane.

If this sample is within a RF receiver coil and M_{xy} is precessing perpendicular to it, an NMR signal will be recorded. The amplitude of the initial signal A_o will depend on the magnitude of the component of M (M_{xy} in the xy plane). The amplitude (A) of this signal decays in an exponential natural log (e) fashion with time, t ($A = A_o e^{-t/T_2}$) as the individual magnetic moments dephase or lose coherence. T_2 relaxation time is the characteristic or average decay time for the process.

Following a 90° RF pulse, the mean vector M is seen to lie along the Y axis (Fig. 5.20). When the RF field is turned off, the proton magnetic moments start to realign with the large external magnetic field B. At any time during realignment, the magnetization M can be considered a vector composed of a transverse component M_{xy} and a longitudinal component M_z. Following the 90° RF pulse, the transverse component of magnetization M_{xy} decays quickly to 0 as the longitudinal component M_z slowly grows to its original value. The rate of decay of the transverse magnetization M_{xy} is exponential with the time constant T_2 transverse relaxation time (Fig. 5.21). The rate of growth of M_z along the longitudinal axis is also exponential with the time constant T_1, the longitudinal relaxation time.

T_2 is a measure of how long the substance maintains the temporary transverse magnetization, which is perpendicular to the external magnetic field. It indicates the relationship between the strength and homogeneity of the external field and the amount of resonance interaction occurring between precessing protons in the tissue. Protons maintaining the transverse magnetization are coherent or wobbling or oscillating in phase about the vertical axis. Phase coherence of the

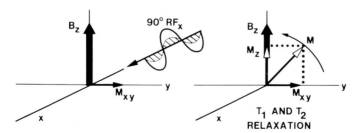

FIG. 5.20. After the 90° RF pulse is terminated, tissue magnetization begins to relax in both the M_{xy} and M_z planes and, at any time after the RF_x pulse, can be thought of as having vector components of M_z and M_{xy}. M_{xy} is lost or relaxes by virtue of the individual proton magnetic moments precessing about the z axis at different rates and therefore losing phase coherence (T_2 relaxation), whereas M_z relaxation occurs by a realignment of M along the z axis (T_1 relaxation). Note: In the static frame of reference M actually spirals upward around the z axis until full relaxation when it again precesses around z.

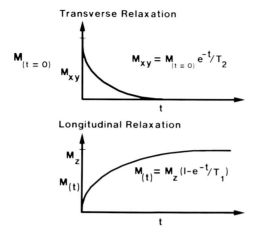

FIG. 5.21. T_2 relaxation is a decay of net magnetization in the M_{xy} plane with an exponential time constant T_2 or transverse relaxation time, whereas longitudinal relaxation along the z axis is an exponential rate of growth of M along the z axis with time constant T_1 or the longitudinal relaxation time.

protons is destroyed by inhomogeneous external magnetic fields resonance flipping of protons precessing at the same frequency and local internal magnetic fields.

Following a FID 90° RF_x pulse (FID) the signal vanishes because the transverse component of the magnetization decays. If the magnetic fields were really homogeneous, the decay constant would be equal to T_2, the transverse relaxation time. This situation is unrealistic, and in practice the magnetic fields generated by magnets have some inhomogeneity. The effective time constant governing signal decay T2* is therefore always shorter than T_2.

The second process affecting the time evolution of the transverse magnetization results from the interactions among the nuclei themselves. Nuclei produce small incremental magnetic fields which also cause dispersal of M_{xy}. This is an intrinsic process, that is, it is independent of instrumental imperfections. It is a random process, governed solely by the random flipping of two neighboring protons which are precessing at the same frequency, or in other words, spin-spin relaxation time T_2. The importance of T2* and T_2 in NMR is that in spin-echo imaging T2*, the incoherence due to external field inhomogeneity, is reversible but T_2 is not reversible.

FREE INDUCTION DECAY

One of the most fundamental examples of a pulsed nuclear magnetic resonance experiment is demonstrated by the free induction decay (FID). An RF pulse at the resonant frequency rotates the M_z vector out of the z direction, and when the pulse is terminated, one observes an oscillating sine wave signal [$\sin(\omega t)$] that decreases in amplitude in exponential fashion with time (e^{-t}/T_2), as shown in Fig 5.22. Essentially, in this example, the amplitude of the signal that corresponds to the number of protons in the tissue is recorded as an oscillating sine wave voltage (beats), and the signal is recorded over the duration in which that signal is emitted. Thus, this is an amplitude versus time plot and is referred to as the free induction decay signal. The FID decays exponentially in a homogeneous external magnetic field. Because the external field is not homogeneous however, it is to be noted that while the free induction signal decays with a time constant $T2*(<T_2)$, the echo amplitude decays with a time constant T_2, the true spin-spin relaxation time.

To state this important principle in a slightly different way, in NMR it is the transverse magnetization, M_{xy}, which is time-dependent and thus according to Faraday's Law of Induction can induce a voltage in a receiver coil. By contrast, the longitudinal magnetization is static and thus does not meet the requirements for magnetic induction. Once the 90° RF_x pulse is removed, the magnetization is subjected to the effect of the static magnetic field (B) only, and thus, precesses about it. During this post-excitation or free precession period, after the radio frequency field has been turned off, the magnetic moment can induce a voltage in a receiver coil, situated in the transverse plane. Since precession occurs at the Larmor frequency, the voltage induced in the coil circuit is of the same frequency. However, the transverse magnetization M_{xy} does not persist. It decays to zero with a characteristic time constant (T_2) and so does the amplitude of the

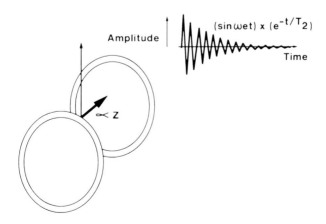

FIG. 5.22. Following an RF pulse, the fundamental NMR signal recorded is a damped amplitude wave that decays with time constant T_2 and is referred to as the free induction decay (FID) and as such represents one of the most fundamental experiments in NMR spectroscopy.

detected voltage (see Fig. 5.22). For this reason, the signal is called free induction decay (FID), manifesting itself as a damped signal oscillation or beats. Because the initial signal amplitude is proportional to the transverse magnetization, which is itself proportional to the number of nuclei excited in a particular voxel of tissue, differences in hydrogen density become discernible in the NMR image.

MOLECULAR PHYSICAL STATE AND T_1 AND T_2

Solid State vs Liquid State NMR

Solids (i.e., cortical bone) have relatively fixed molecules with relatively fixed magnetic fields, and these cause significant local variations in the value of the magnetic field around any given proton.

In a liquid (i.e., soft tissue) the local magnetic fields from neighboring molecules fluctuate rapidly as the molecules move about, and the end result contributes little to the net magnetic field at any point.

T_1 is much longer for solids than for liquids. In an external magnetic field, as we have seen previously, protons align parallel and antiparallel with the imposed magnetic field. This process of alignment occurs by molecular thermal interaction, i.e., molecules within the sample collide or interact with each other, thus transferring energy. In solids (which can be thought of in general as crystalline lattices), molecules are relatively fixed and do not collide frequently, whereas in liquids molecules are free to collide with each other, thereby transferring energy and facilitating proton realignment in the field. As an analogy, the transfer of energy to the lattice can be thought of in terms of two sailors trying to jump onto a dock from their respective boats, one of which has been left on the land by the receding tide and the other which is freely floating in the water. As the two jump, the sailor in the water transfers much of his energy to the boat, which moves easily in the liquid water lattice, and the sailor quickly realigns by falling into the water, whereas the sailor jumping from the landlocked boat retains most of his energy and remains aligned by landing upright on the pier successfully (Fig. 5.23). T_1 is also called *spin-* (spinning proton) *lattice* (physical matrix of the molecule in the sample) *relaxation*. As we have seen previously, it is often called *longitudinal relaxation* because of the longitudinal orientation with the z axis (Table 5.1).

T_2 is much shorter for solids than liquids. In solids the molecular structure tends to be fixed, and their associated magnetic fields are fixed as well. These local inhomogeneities are significant and cause

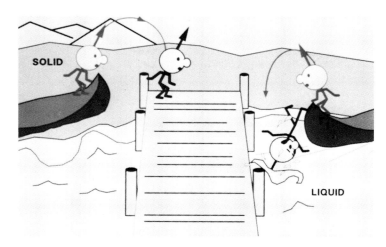

FIG. 5.23. The physical state has a profound effect on the relaxation times. T_1 relaxation occurs by the exchange of thermal energy between molecules. Protons in a solid state are able to retain most of their energy and remain aligned (land upright on the dock) but protons in the liquid state quickly transfer much of their energy to the water and lose alignment (landing upside down in the water). T_1 relaxation is much faster in liquids than in solids for similar reasons: in liquids thermal energy transfer from the protons to the surrounding molecules occurs much more quickly because the molecules are freer to move and collide with each other and they thus change alignment more quickly.

significant intermagnetic field effects, especially when the opposing magnetic fields are pointed in the opposite or unaligned direction. Thus, the magnetic-magnetic or, in NMR parlance, the spin-spin interaction, is quite significant in solids and T_2 is very short. In a liquid, however, molecules are free to move rapidly, and thus their net local magnetization averages very quickly to zero and contributes little so that magnetic-magnetic, or spin-spin, interactions are not very significant. Consequently, for liquids the internal fields are weaker, and T_2 encounters less dephasing magnetic influence, and the T_2 time constant is longer. Again, as the transverse M_{xy} component decays, the longitudinal component is growing at a rate T_1 due to thermal collisions. Therefore, T_2 is often referred to as the transverse (transverse to the external magnetic field) spin-spin (magnetic field to magnetic field interaction) relaxation time (see Table 5.1).

Since solid tissues and other solid specimens have fixed static internal magnetic fields that cause variation in the local magnetic field, there are local variations in the proton resonant frequency, and the FID for solids is composed of many sine waves of differing frequen-

TABLE 5.1. T_1 and T_2 spin-lattice relaxation

| Relaxation process | | Liquid state | | Solid state |
		Typical value[a] for H_2O at 4 MHz	Typical value[a] for in vivo soft tissue at 4 MHz (large molecules)	Bone, crystals, etc.
T_1 Spin-lattice relaxation (Molecular-Thermal)	Longitudinal	2,700 msec	600 msec	Very long
T_2 Spin-spin relaxation (Magnetic-Magnetic)	Transverse	2,700 msec	30 msec	Very short

[a] T_1 and T_2 for a proton nucleus vary as a function of temperature, pH, resonant frequency and chemical composition. These values are relative (ref. 31).

cies. Since they quickly get out of phase, the corresponding FID curve is short (short T_2). For pure liquids the effect of internal magnetic fields is much less, and the proton resonant frequency is determined almost entirely by the external magnetic field. Thus, there is only one local resonant frequency shared by all the protons in the excited region. They remain in phase, and therefore, the FID for liquids is long, and the curve can be represented by one sine wave— or by superimposed sine waves of almost the same frequency. For solids having an FID composed of sine waves of many frequencies, the frequency spectrum is broad. For liquids the range of frequencies (or the width of frequency spectrum) is quite narrow. This is demonstrated in Fig. 5.24 where the amplitude of the sine waves that make up the FID is plotted against the respective frequency. The resultant peak is broad based for solids and narrow for liquids.

Liquid State NMR: Dissolved Small Molecules vs Large Molecules

With the exception of cortical bone, calculi or metallic clips most body tissues can be thought of as liquids with various sized molecules dissolved or suspended within them. Cerebral spinal fluid is an example of a liquid with very small molecules, such as salts, dissolved within it. Small molecules tumble or move very rapidly in pure liquid such as cerebral spinal fluid and this rate of movement or tumbling is much higher than the Larmor frequencies used in nuclear magnetic resonance imaging. The frequency difference does not allow an efficient exchange of energy. Therefore, relaxation times (i.e., T_1) are very long in pure liquids or liquids which have small molecules within them. Conversely, most body tissues have much larger molecular sizes associated with the proteins, fats, and complex sugars which make up their parencyma and relaxation times are much shorter. This occurs because with increasing size larger molecules tumble or oscillate more slowly. At some point frequencies which are much closer to the Larmor frequencies used in NMR imaging are obtained which in turn results in resonance and more efficient energy transfer and faster relaxation times. Beyond this size T_1 again lengthens. The shorter relaxation times in white matter when compared to gray matter are due to the hydrogen protons being bound to the much larger myelin molecules in white matter.

The representation of the FID curve by its component frequencies amounts to transforming the amplitude versus time information of the FID into a plot of amplitude versus frequency. This is usually accomplished by using a Fourier transform, named after its originator,

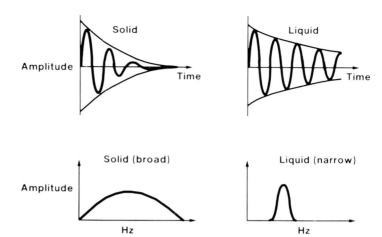

FIG. 5.24. Physical state has a significant effect on T_2 relaxation time. T_2 relaxation occurs by magnetic interaction of protons. Solids have fixed internal magnetic fields that cause variation in the local magnetic field, and therefore, precessing protons rapidly dephase and the free induction decay (FID) for solids is composed of many sine waves of differing (broad) frequency and the T_2 relaxation time is short. In liquids internal magnetic fields are not static, and the internal fields quickly sum to zero, having much less effect on the precessing protons. Therefore, the frequency band of precessing protons is narrow and the relaxation time is long. These are significant considerations because variation in relaxation time have a significant effect on NMR image quality.

French mathematician Jean Baptiste Fourier (Digital Fourier Transform—DFT) (Fig. 5.25).

As we shall see later in the chapter on NMR imaging (Chapter 6), Fourier transformation is important in image reconstruction of magnetic resonance. It is basically a method to convert a complex waveform expressed in amplitude range over a given period of time (time domain) to the component frequencies of that waveform in an amplitude versus frequency plot (frequency domain). In the frequency domain in NMR spectroscopy, a narrow spectral line with a narrow peak and long tail is referred to as a *Lorentzian line*. In actual application, all of the frequencies coming from an excited sample or tissue are measured simultaneously, and the information is sent to a computer that analyzes the signal strength at each of the freqencies of interest. This frequency analysis is carried out by a classical mathematical maneuver, the Fourier transform. The formal Fourier transform is an expensive use of computer time, and an abbreviated form called the *fast Fourier transform* is universally used. It is this transformation that is the basis of the computed image reconstruction in all of the modern CT techniques.

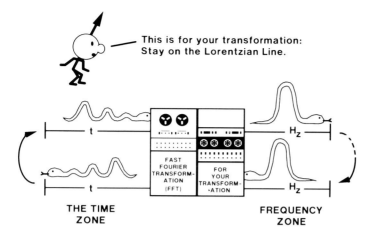

FIG. 5.25. In NMR image reconstruction it is important to change the radio wave NMR signal from an amplitude vs time display (time zone) to an amplitude vs frequency display (frequency domain) because the frequency is used to locate the signal in space, whereas the amplitude is used to determine the number of protons present in that space. This transformation is performed using a sophisticated computer algorithm called the *Fourier transformation* (FT). Using the FT is analogous to separating white light into its color components with a prism.

INVERSION-RECOVERY TECHNIQUE

An extension of this discussion suggests that most magnetic resonance experiments divide naturally into two periods: periods of excitation and periods of emission or "listening" in which the RF signal from the sample is observed (Fig. 5.26). If this delay time is made too short, however, there is a decrease in initial amplitude, A_o, observed in the subsequent experiment. This happens because insufficient time is allowed for longitudinal relaxation, and M_z is not fully recovered to the equilibrium value. This provides a useful technique for evaluating T_1 with a preparative excitation technique as discussed below.

Measurement of T_1

As noted above, by adjusting the length of the RF pulse, we achieved a 90° RF_x that gave the maximum possible signal amplitude, A_o, in the xy plane (M_{xy}). By doubling the length (2 90° RF_x), we can rotate M through 180° or, in fact, any angle α desired (αRF). The magnitude of the longitudinal net magnetization M_z then varies as a function of time in an exponential fashion with the rate constant $1/T_1$.

Due to the way NMR scanners are configured, longitudinal relaxation

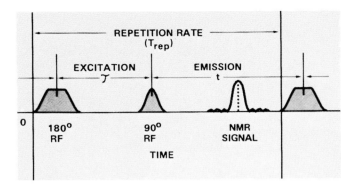

FIG. 5.26. Many imaging schemes are used in NMR scanning. However, these experiments naturally divide into two periods: a period of excitation or irradiation of the tissue with RF pulses and a period during which the RF coils are tuned to listen for the emitted NMR signal. The period of time between the sets of tissue irradiation is referred to as the repetition rate (T_{rep} or TR).

along the z axis cannot be observed directly. Only vectors moving perpendicular to the RF coil will generate an NMR signal. Thus, in practice, to observe the relaxation along the z axis, a second 90° RF pulse needs to be applied to the sample during recovery (Fig. 5.26). One can measure the actual time required for longitudinal relaxation along the z axis by following the 180° pulse with variably spaced 90° pulses, and where a maximal signal is recorded after the last 90° pulse, complete relaxation can be assumed to have occurred. This method is called *inversion recovery* (i.e., inversion of the magnetization from M_z to M_{-z}, and then subsequent recovery or relaxation). In practice, multiple averages are taken for each 180° to 90° interval. However, the time between pulse pairs or the repetition rate is kept long to allow total recovery of the tissue between RF excitation. This method is more sensitive than saturation recovery (90° RF_x) to differences in T_1.

The inversion-recovery technique is used in some magnetic resonance imaging experiments to give an evaluation of T_1 or at least a T_1 weighting of the image. In addition, there are other preparative excitation sequences using alternative pulsing arrangements to deliver other types of magnetic resonance data as we shall see in the section on imaging.

SPIN-ECHO TECHNIQUE

Many explanations of the spin-echo technique use the rotating frame of reference, which rotates with the precessing nuclear moments to study the relative magnetic vector changes. In some cases the motion of the net magnetization is easier to understand. In some respects it is confusing, and in this section T_2 will be discussed using a static frame of reference. However, those readers going on to other texts should be sure to determine whether or not the author is discussing the spin-echo technique using the rotating frame or static frame of reference approach.

In Chapter 4 we discussed the tendency of tops in a gravitational field to wobble or precess around the gravitational field. Similarly, ensembles of protons with magnetic moments tend to align with and precess around an externally applied static magnetic field.

As opposed to the free induction decay, the spin-echo is an RF signal that returns (echoes) after a delay. The amplitude of the spin-echo is directly related to the number of protons in the tissue irradiated and how well they remain in phase (T_2). The frequency of the spin-echo indicates the strength of the local magnetic field determined by the external gradient, and the form of the echo display is a mirror image of the free induction decay.

The spin-echo is produced by first exposing the tissue that has been placed in a static external magnetic field to a 90° RF pulse along the x axis (90° RF_x). The magnetization M of the excited volume that was pointing along the z axis is not rotated 90° so that it points along the y axis. After the 90° RF_x pulse, M precesses about the z axis at the same precessional frequency ω. Small variations in the external magnetic field in the excited tissue cause some protons to experience slightly stronger and some slightly weaker magnetic fields. Those in the stronger local magnetic fields, M_h, are going to precess at a slightly higher frequency than those in the weaker local magnetic field, M_t. As the protons lose coherence or phase, those in the weaker field (M_t) will move more slowly and lag behind those experiencing a slightly higher field with magnetization (M_h). After an interval (τ) following 90° RF_x, the sample is exposed to a 180° pulse from the RF_x coil that causes a further 180° rotation about the x axis. This results in the y component of the magnetization vector changing sign while the x component is unaffected. Following this 180° RF_x, vectors M_h and M_t continue to precess in the counter-clockwise direction. However, the effect of the 180° pulse is such that the slower precessing vectors are now in front of the faster precessing vectors, and the faster overtake the slower with a crescendo-decrescendo echo recorded as the spin-echo with the vectors coming into and then losing coherence. This signal height is proportional to the proton density and T_2 and is called the *spin-echo*.

We can appreciate this relationship somewhat better if we shift our conventional frame of reference and take a position high on the z axis and look down at the xy plane. The faster moving vectors can be represented by those attached to the hare (M_h) and slower by those attached to the tortoise (M_t). The longer the two are allowed to "race" the farther ahead the hare will be. If we were to pick up the vector of the tortoise and the hare, such that their relative position along the y axis was the same but the tortoise was now ahead of the hare at some point, the hare would catch up with the tortoise and the two vectors would be coherent again for a short period of time. At this point the amplitude along the y axis would be the greatest, and a signal would be recorded. Since the progress of the faster hare is overtaking and then passing that of the tortoise, there is an ascending signal to maximum coherence and a descending signal giving a mirror-image configuration (Fig. 5.27). In magnetic resonance imaging, this effect of changing the position of the tortoise and the hare is achieved by a 180° RF_x pulse. This can be repeated as many times as is necessary for adequate imaging.

In summary, the spin-echo is produced by a 90° RF pulse followed by a 180° RF pulse. The FID resulting from saturation-recovery or inversion-recovery sequences can also be converted to a spin-echo if a 180° pulse follows the last 90° pulse. The strength of the spin-echo depends on hydrogen density and T_2. T_1 can be distinguished by variations of the time between pulse pairs (i.e., TR, the repetition rate).

Measurement of T_2

The measurement of T_2 using the spin-echo technique was first proposed by Hahn (*Physics Review*, 80:580, 1950), using the 90°, τ, 180° sequence, and the subsequent observation at a time 2τ of a free induction "echo." After the 90° RF_x pulse, the precessional frequencies are in phase but very quickly begin to fan out as some of the nuclei precess faster than others. At a time τ after the 90° pulse, a 180° pulse is applied as we have seen in the spin-echo sequence, which has the effect of placing the more rapidly precessing magnetic moments behind the slower. At a time 2τ, all the individual magnetic moments come into phase and the continuing movement causes them again to lose phase coherence. The reshaping of the fanned out magnetic moments (M) causes a free induction signal to build to a maximum at 2τ. If transverse relaxation did not occur, the echo amplitude might be just as large as the initial value of the free induction following the 90° pulse, but some magnetic moment (M) coherence decreases during the time 2τ because of the natural process responsible

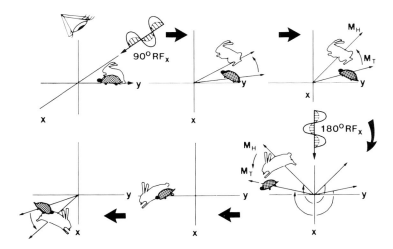

FIG. 5.27. The NMR signal in the spin-echo technique is produced due to the fact that following the 90° RF_x pulse, all proton magnetic moments are inphase in the xy plane, but subsequently due to local variations in the magnetic field, some of the protons precess faster (M_h) than others (M_t). If, however, a subsequent 180° RF_x pulse is broadcast into the sample, the individual magnetic moments undergo a 180° rotation about or around the x axis, which results in the faster precessing magnetic moments being behind the slower ones. A crescendo-decrescendo (echo) signal is produced as these faster magnetic moments overtake, stay briefly in phase with, and then pass beyond the slower magnetic moments. The time required for this phase coherence to be reestablished is exactly equal to the elapsed time between the 90° RF_x and the 180° RF_x pulse. This tissue irradiation can be repeated several times; however, coherence of the NMR signal in spin-echo technique is lost due to two processes: (1) Due to inhomogeneities in the fluctuating internal field of the substance produced by magnetic dipoles in the nuclei and resonance spin-spin flipping and this loss cannot be reconstituted. Therefore, over time the NMR spin-echo signal decreases in intensity. (2) Due to inhomogeneities in the external magnetic field. Since the phase in coherence induced by the external magnetic field is constant, it can be reconstituted, R. To summarize, transverse magnetization is lost by two processes rapidly due to nonuniformity in the external magnetic field produced by the NMR scanner **(B)**, (designated T_2^*) and more slowly due to internal field nonuniformity due to characteristics of the tissue (designated T_2). Inhomogeneity in the external field (T_2^*) determines the width of the spin-echo and T_2 determines the height of successive echos.

for transverse relaxation in the time T_2. Thus, the echo amplitude depends on T_2, and for a sample with only a single resonant frequency, T_2 may in principle be determined from a plot of peak echo amplitude as a function of τ. In the more general case, however, since the echo is just 2 FIDs back-to-back, Fourier transformation of half the echo results in a spectrum with line heights dependent on their individual T_2s. As in the measurement of T_1 by the 180° RF_x τ 90° RF_x method, it is necessary to carry out a separate pulse sequence for each value of τ and to wait between pulse sequences and allow adequate time (at least 5 × T_1) for restoration of equilibrium.

The spin-echo technique is limited in its range of applicability because of the effect of molecular diffusion. The precise refocusing of all precessing magnetic moments (M) is dependent on each nucleus remaining in a constant magnetic field during the time of the experiment. If diffusion causes nuclei to move from one part of an inhomogeneous field to another, the echo amplitude is reduced. Diffusion coefficients are thus readily measured by spin-echo technique.

The Carr and Purcell method (17) for measuring T_2 is an improvement on the simple spin-echo technique. This method uses 180° pulses that are applied at τ, 2τ, 3τ, 5τ, etc., to form echoes at 2τ, 4τ, 6τ, etc. The height of the echoes is more accurate because many such echoes may be formed in short time intervals to preclude appreciable diffusion. Actually, small mis-settings of pulse would cause cumulative errors that can be overcome by a shift in RF phase, which is the Meiboom and Gill method.

Chapter 6

Magnetic Resonance Imaging (MRI)

IMAGING METHODS IN NUCLEAR MAGNETIC RESONANCE

Although we are only going to deal with a few examples of the imaging methods commonly used in magnetic resonance imaging, the reader should be aware that there are a large number of options for generating images in terms of manipulating field gradients and RF pulses, and there are an equally large number of options in terms of the method of image reconstruction (see Appendix). For those interested in the general spectrum of NMR imaging options, however, the following list should suffice:

1. Direct dimensional (D) imaging
2. Echo-planar
3. Field focusing nuclear magnetic resonance (FONAR)
4. Fourier zeugmatography (Phase and Frequency Shifts)
5. Rotating-frame zeugmatography (Flip Angle Variation)
6. Selective irradiation
7. Sensitive-region (oscillating field) method—plane, line, point

Imaging techniques in NMR can be classified in four general technique categories depending on the actual volume of tissue that is excited or irradiated and from which the signal is received to make an image. Depending on how the NMR scanner is configured, the excited or irradiated volume can be a single point, a line, a plane, or a large volume of tissue. All of these methods produce images that are ultimately resolved into single points or voxels, but the way these points are defined and irradiated or excited in the imaging sequence varies. The single-point technique defines the points in the image by exciting and measuring points or voxels one at a time. Three-dimensional reconstruction methods repeatedly excite and measure and then using various computer algorithms, calculates the signal contributed by each point or voxel in the objects. The type of imaging method used has important consequences for the quality of the ultimate NMR image. One of the difficulties in NMR imaging is the large noise background relative to the NMR signal (signal-to-noise ratio). The signal-to-noise ratio depends on a variety of factors including strength of the magnetic field, total volume of the room temperature magnet bore, the imaging technique used, and the excitation volume. Most of the intrinsic noise in the NMR scanning system is determined by the NMR instrument itself, but it is important to realize that the value of signal-to-noise ratio in the instrument is not equivalent to the signal-to-noise ratio in the following image. Since the excitation of larger volumes produces larger NMR signals and the noise level is determined by the scanner, improvement in signal-to-noise ratio results when the whole volume excitation methods are employed. On the other hand, as the size of the resolution volume increases with respect to the object size, blurring will decrease contrast in the ultimate image. Thus, when a very small object is scanned with a relatively large resolution volume, although signal-to-noise increases for the instrument, blurring will decrease contrast in that ultimate image. As we shall see shortly, the FID signal provides a stronger signal than do pulse echoes in the spin-echo technique, thus yielding an improved signal-to-noise ratio for the instrument. However, in this imaging sequence, T_2 information and the contrast it provides is lost. The spin-echo technique may actually provide a higher signal-to-noise ratio in the ultimate image by enhancing contrast between adjacent organs with different T_2 relaxation times.

Essentially, the imaging techniques used in NMR involve a series of options regarding the sequencing of either 90° RF or 180° RF pulses and the timing or sequencing of the series of sets of pulses (repetition rate). The options are used to spatially encode and determine different characteristics of tissue, i.e., proton density, T_1 and T_2 relaxation times. The strategies are designed primarily to elicit some aspect of the NMR signal in preference to others with an eye toward a more accurate diagnosis or better resolution (Figs. 6.1 to 6.7).

Inversion recovery and spin-echo are the two most commonly employed imaging methods in use today. Another method that is commonly used in spectroscopy is called the *steady-state free precession* or *continuous wave* method. In this NMR technique, the magnetic field is periodically tipped by closely pulsed RF excitations. These pulses are short with respect to the T_1 of the sample being irradiated, and in this method the FID from each pulse merges with the previous pulse and forms a continuous NMR signal. A continuous signal has the advantage of providing a steady rather than transient source of energy. However, the nuclei are never allowed to return to equilib-

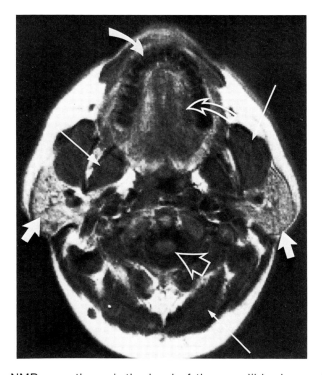

FIG. 6.1. An NMR scan through the level of the mandible demonstrating the excellent image quality obtainable from NMR scanning systems operating at the relatively high strength of 5 KG. Note the white subcutaneous fat, muscles (*long arrows*), teeth (*solid curved arrow*), spinal cord (*open arrowhead*), tongue (*open curved arrow*), and parotid glands (*solid arrows*).

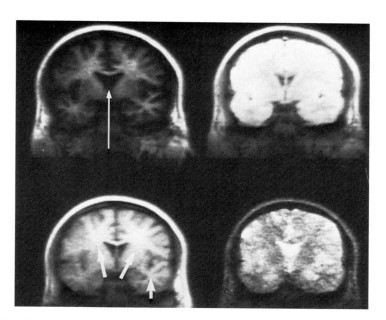

FIG. 6.2. Coronal NMR scans at the level of the lateral ventricle demonstrating the effect of different pulse sequences on the NMR image. A relatively short (0.5 sec, *lower left*) and a relatively long (2.0 sec, *upper right*) saturation-recovery interpulse interval is compared with an inversion-recovery (*upper left*) and spin-echo technique images (*lower right*). Note the marked changes in gray and white matter contrast enhancement and the changes in cerebral spinal fluid NMR signal intensity in the lateral ventricles on the various images. The 0.5-sec saturation-recovery image (*lower left*) demonstrates the white matter as white (*short arrows*) because of the shorter T_1 in white matter as opposed to gray matter. Shorter relaxation times (T_1 and T_2) in white matter are due to the protons being bound to large molecules in the myelin in the white matter, which promotes faster relaxation. When the pulse interval greatly exceeds T_1 relaxation (2.0 sec, *upper right*), the image tends to reflect proton density distribution, and white and gray matter show a decrease in contrast resolution. The inversion-recovery image (*upper left*) is also T_1 weighted and further accentuates the T_1 differences between white (short T_1) and gray (longer T_1) matter. CSF in this image appears black because the T_1 of CSF is very long due to the large preponderance of very small molecules that tumble or move much more rapidly than the Larmor frequency and therefore do not exchange energy efficiently (i.e., prolonged relaxation times). By comparison, the spin-echo image (*lower right*) emphasizes T_2 differences between tissues, and the most striking phenomenon here is the increased NMR signal from the cerebral spinal fluid in the ventricles (white); this is due to the very prolonged T_2 relaxation time of CSF when compared to surrounding brain tissue. Also note the reversal between white and gray matter in that white matter has a lower (darker) NMR signal reflecting the faster T_2 relaxation in white matter as opposed to gray matter. (Copyright Technicare Corporation. NMR image provided by courtesy of Technicare Corporation.)

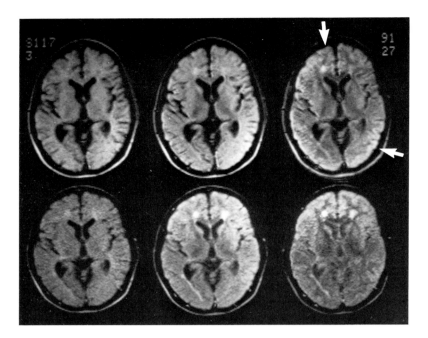

FIG. 6.3. A series of NMR scans obtained utilizing the spin-echo technique and a two echo protocol, including images obtained from the first echo (28 msec, *top row*) and the second echo (56 msec, *bottom row*) and a 0.5-, 1.0- or 1.5-sec rep rate (*left to right*). In this imaging sequence, the effect of utilizing the first or second spin-echo to achieve T_2 weighting can be gained by comparing images in the top row with images in the bottom row. The effect of changing the rep rate to introduce T_1 weighting can be gained by scanning each row from left to right. Those tissues with the longest T_1 relaxation times will have the most intense NMR signal (white) on the right. For any given T_1 weighting, the greatest contrast enhancement between tissues with variable T_2 relaxation times will be seen on the bottom row as compared to the image above it. Note in the top row, as one moves from left to right, the relative increase in NMR signal obtained from gray matter, which is most pronounced in the upper right-hand image (the longest rep rate of 1.5 sec that allows full relaxation from the relatively long T_1 of gray matter and therefore a maximal NMR signal from it, *arrows*). Note also the relative increase in NMR signal obtained from the CSF and the ventricles comparing the upper right (1.5-sec rep rate and 28-msec interpulse interval) and lower right (1.5-sec rep rate and 56-msec interpulse interval). The longer interpulse interval of the lower right image allows the longer T_2 relaxation time of the CSF and the ventricles to increase the CSF NMR signal, and in this particular imaging method, the CSF has become nearly iso-dense with the surrounding white matter. In addition, note that due to similar T_2 weighting, the contrast resolution between gray and white matter has been preserved. T_2 weighting in this case has taken advantage of the fact that T_2 relaxation in gray matter is approximately 20% longer than that of white matter, and therefore the longer interpulse echo time of 56 msec has allowed further accentuation of gray-white contrast resolution. Although actual relaxation time measurements are instrument dependent, the best current estimate for T_2 relaxation is 80 msec for white matter and 100 msec for gray matter. (NMR image courtesy of University of California, San Francisco Radiologic Imaging Laboratory.)

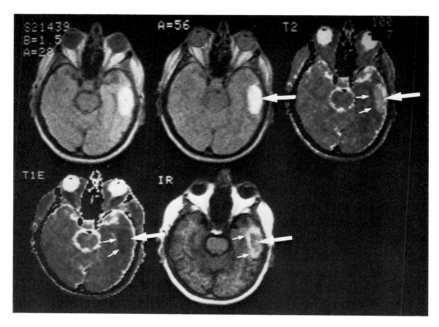

FIG. 6.4. A series of NMR scans obtained at the same level in a patient with a left temporal lobe hematoma, utilizing the following imaging techniques: *upper left*—1.5-sec rep rate/28-msec echo; *top row, middle*—1.5-sec rep rate/56-msec echo; *top, right*—calculated T_2 image; *bottom, left*—calculated T_1 image; and *bottom, right*—inversion-recovery image. Note that the characteristic NMR appearance of cerebral hemorrhage in the rim of the hemorrhage has a shortened relaxation time (*short arrows*), whereas the central portion of the hemorrhage demonstrates a lengthening of the relaxation times (*long arrows*). The prolongation of relaxation times in the central portion of the hemorrhage is consistent with the pathologic findings of an increase in the amount of liquification in aging hemorrhages as demonstrated by Enzmann et al., in 1982. These characteristic differential zones of cerebral hemorrhage are well demonstrated in the calculated T_2 and T_1 images as well as in the inversion-recovery image. (NMR image provided courtesy of the University of California San Francisco Radiologic Imaging Laboratory.)

rium with the main field, and thus, the NMR signal is reduced but the signal-to-noise ratio is relatively high because it can have a very long duration.

STANDARDIZED IMAGING SEQUENCE

NMR experiments or imaging methods can be thought of in terms of two periods. A period of tissue excitation or preparation and a

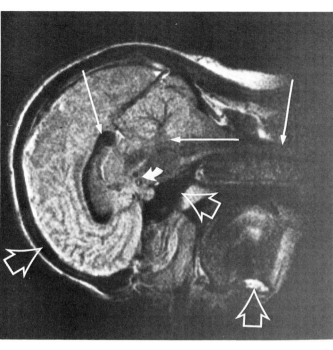

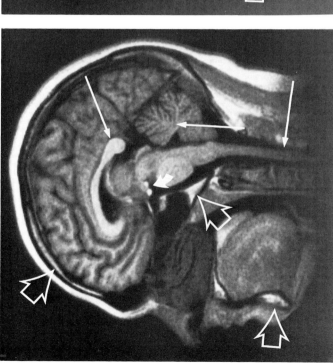

FIG. 6.5. Midline sagittal NMR images recorded on a 0.3-T imaging system using an inversion-recovery technique with 1-sec pulse sequence duration and T_2 information was added by introducing two 180° spin-echo pulses at 200- (*left*) and 500- (*right*) msec interpulse delays. The images were acquired using a 256 × 256 matrix and 9-mm slices. Note that in this case the additional weighting of T_2 information in the figure on the right has decreased the clarity of the image and specifically converted white matter and spinal cord from a white to black signal (*long arrows*), decreased the signal from bone marrow (*open arrows*). (NMR image provided courtesy of the General Electric Co.)

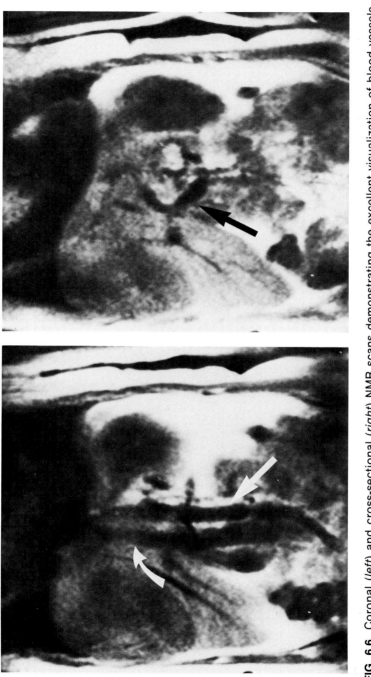

FIG. 6.6. Coronal (*left*) and cross-sectional (*right*) NMR scans demonstrating the excellent visualization of blood vessels, i.e., aorta (*straight white arrow*), inferior vena cava (*curved arrow*), and portal vein (*black arrow*), due to the fact that little NMR signal is obtained from moving structures such as the intravascular blood in this case (0.3-T field strength, 1-cm slice thickness). (Copyright Technicare Corporation. NMR image provided by courtesy of Technicare Corporation.)

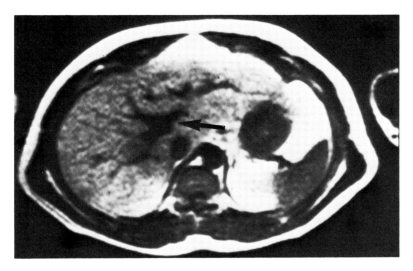

FIG. 6.6. continued.

period of emission of the absorbed excitation or a period of listening. The methods by which these parameters are manipulated are by varying the pulse sequences as follows:

Pulse sequences: Sets of RF (and/or gradient) magnetic field pulses and time spacings between these pulses; used in conjunction with gradient magnetic fields and NMR signal reception to produce NMR images.

Interpulse times: Times between successive RF pulses used in pulse sequences. Particularly important are the inversion time (T_I) in inversion recovery and the time between a 90° pulse and subsequent 180° pulse to produce a spin echo. This interval will be approximately one half the spin echo time (TE). The time between repetitions of pulse sequences is the repetition time (TR) (see Appendix I, III).

IMAGE QUALITY: THE EFFECT OF PULSE SEQUENCE AND VARIATIONS IN T_1 AND T_2

The NMR signal on which the NMR image is based increases (becomes whiter in the gray-scale NMR image) with magnetic field strength and with:

↑ Proton density
↓ T_1
↑ T_2
↓ Motion (flow)

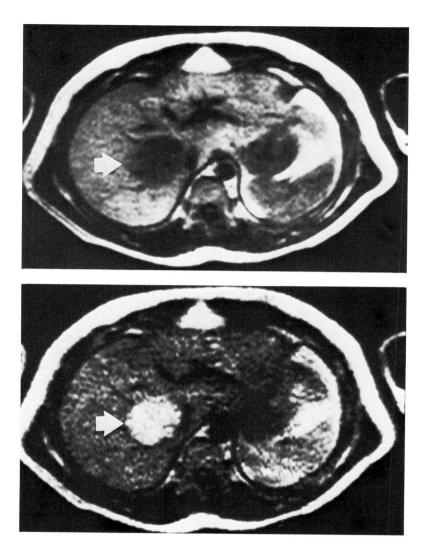

FIG. 6.7. Cross-sectional NMR scans of a patient with an hepatic metastasis (*arrow*) demonstrating the improved contrast resolution of an imaging technique devoid of spin-echo information (*top,* saturation recovery) and one spin-echo (*bottom*) containing T_2 information. Note that although there is a wide variation, in general, neoplasms show an increase in both T_1 and T_2 relaxation times. This case demonstrates this phenomenon in that the saturation-recovery T_1 weighted image demonstrates the hepatic neoplasm as a decreased (black) NMR signal reflecting the prolonged T_1 of the neoplasm relative to the surrounding hepatic tissue. Conversely, in the spin-echo image, the lengthened T_2 of the neoplasm is revealed as a white lesion reflecting the T_2 weighting of the spin-echo techniques that exploit prolongation of T_2 relaxation. (Copyright Technicare Corporation. NMR image provided by courtesy of Technicare Corporation and the University Hospitals of Cleveland.)

The NMR image is extremely dependent on the techniques employed in administering the various RF frequency pulses because of these relationships. Appropriately applied, RF pulse sequences can increase the contrast between tissues by exploiting differences between their relaxation times. If we consider adjusting the sequence by shortening the rep rate, we begin to decrease the signal coming from those tissues with a longer T_1, while those with shorter T_1s (i.e., those T_1s shorter than the rep rate) maintain their signal intensity. In spin-echo technique, by lengthening the interpulse interval, although the spin-echo amplitudes of all tissues decline, those with longer T_2s maintain their signal intensity, whereas short T_2 signal intensities fall off rapidly. The absolute measurement of T_1 and T_2 relaxation times is very dependent on the equipment utilized; however, as a general approximation, if we compare muscle and fat, the respective T_1 and T_2 values for muscle are 0.7 sec-T_1 and 32 msec-T_2 and for fat, 0.3 sec-T_1 and 50 msec-T_2. As we adjust the NMR imaging instrumentation, fat will become brighter (whiter) when compared to muscle with a short rep rate (TR) interval (due to the short T_1) and lengthening, the interpulse interval (TE) (due to the long T_2). Utilizing these techniques, it is possible to calculate T_1 and T_2 images and to assign a gray scale value to the tissues according to T_1 or T_2. It is important to remember that in NMR imaging, varying the T_1 and T_2 parameters can also selectively enhance the contrast between tissues. In the comparison of fat and muscle, lengthening the T_2 parameter will decrease the absolute T_2 signal intensities, but the contrast between tissues will increase. This is important because the signal-to-noise ratio, which is contrast dependent, may be maximized by the appropriate parameter selection. Thus, obtaining NMR images at several instrument T_1 and T_2 settings is advisable because pathological lesions may blend their densities with surrounding normal tissues and may be missed if only one setting is utilized (Fig. 6.3).

NORMAL AND ABNORMAL TISSUES, RELAXATION TIMES, AND IMAGE CONTRAST

When conceptualizing NMR imaging of normal and pathological conditions, it may be helpful to think of the body as basically "soup" with the exception of bones, calculi, metallic surgical clips, etc.

NMR cross-sectional images produced from FID experiments are essentially density maps of the protons contained in tissue in the form of free or bound water and lipid molecules. By adding the relaxation time information to the NMR scan image we can enrich the information within the image and at times greatly increase the contrast differences between tissues. The image is thus based on both proton density and relaxation time information reflecting the way the molecules move within the tissue.

Relaxation in tissue (both T_1 and T_2) occurs because of the intrinsic magnetic fields caused by magnetic dipoles, like those associated with protons, which move (i.e. translate, rotate, and tumble) and thereby create local inhomogeneous magnetic interactions. If these intrinsic fields oscillate at the Larmor frequency, energy is exchanged and transitions are induced. The determining factor is thus frequency or the rate at which molecules move in tissue. Small molecules, inorganic salts, and water tend to reorient at rates much higher than the Larmor frequency, leading to relatively inefficient relaxation (long T_1 and T_2). Larger molecules lipid, fat, and protein move more slowly due to their larger inertia and increased friction with neighboring molecules. As their rate of movement passes the Larmor frequency, more efficient energy exchange and faster relaxation (short T_1 and T_2) occurs. Because of molecular size and motion, water protons relax more slowly than the protons in large lipid molecules such as myelin. Both T_1 and T_2 therefore are characteristically shorter in white matter than in gray matter because the former contains a larger percentage of faster-relaxing lipid protons. Somewhat surprisingly T_1 and T_2 differences have also been observed in tissue with comparable water content. This is believed to be due to differing viscosity and paramagnetic species.

Cerebral spinal fluid has prolonged relaxation time (T_1 and T_2) because it is a pure liquid. White matter has more large myelin molecules. Free water protons have longer relaxation times than bound water because they move faster and don't exchange energy very well. Disease states are often associated with increased water (i.e., edema) and this increase in water, in general, increases relaxation times (T_1 and T_2). Although we shall deal with this subject in greater depth in Chapter 8, paramagnetic contrast agents cause a decrease in relaxation times (T_1 and T_2).

Thus, many conditions tend to cause similar changes in both T_1 and T_2, but T_1 and T_2 are inversely related to image contrast. In other words, a decrease in T_1 increases the NMR signal and potentially its contrast enhancement whereas the simultaneous decrease in T_2 decreases T_2 contrast resolution between tissues, and vice versa. Under these conditions it would be very important to select an imaging method which emphasized T_1 and not T_2 in the final image. Conversely, since we have opposed influences on the image it would also be possible to pick an imaging method which included both T_1 and

T_2 and completely obscure contrast differences. Relaxation times can be used to characterize lesions with NMR (Fig. 6.10). In addition spin-echo information (T_2 weighting) can be added to inversion recovery methods to obtain additional information (Fig. 6.11). In fact all pulse sequences use a 180° spin-echo pulse to get the NMR FID signal away from the "ringing" induced in the RF antenna by the strong 180° inversion pulse.

T_1

In actual NMR imaging, the adjustment of the RF pulses that separate the two periods of excitation and emmission can have an important impact on the quality and diagnostic utility of the NMR image. Following the 90° pulse in FID or inversion recovery, if the rep rate is made too short relative to the length of T_1, there will be a decrease in the initial signal amplitude observed (Fig. 6.8). This occurs because insufficient time is allowed for longitudinal relaxation and M_z is not fully recovered to the equilibrium value. From this perspective two tissues being scanned using inversion recovery and

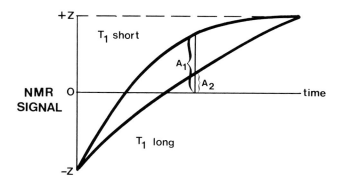

FIG. 6.8. The repetition rate or interpulse interval has a marked effect on the NMR signal obtained from two tissues with varying T_1 relaxation times. A tissue with a short T_1 will have a maximum amplitude (A_1); however, a tissue with a T_1 that is longer will result in a much reduced amplitude (A_2). This effect is seen in an NMR image as a decrease in NMR signal or a shift toward the black end of the gray scale. (See Figs. 6.3 to 6.5.)

a fixed 90° RF$_x$ repetition rate but with markedly different T$_1$ values would have different NMR signals—a very intense signal if the T$_1$ were short and a somewhat less intense signal if T$_1$ in the second tissue was relatively longer.

This principle can be exploited by NMR imaging technology to measure actually the length of T$_1$ in a given sample by adjusting the rep rate when TR is long relative to T$_1$, a maximum signal amplitude is obtained, i.e., A$_1$ in Fig. 6.1. However, if we shorten the T rep and do not allow complete relaxation, we notice a decrease in the initial signal amplitude of the ensuing FID (A$_2$ in Fig. 6.8). If we were to continue this process until no signal was obtained, i.e., A$_n$ = 0, then we would have, by comparing all of the observed values, a good estimate of the exact length of T$_1$.

Inversion-recovery images depend on hydrogen density, flow, and T$_1$, but there is little contribution from T$_2$. In general, the brightest portions of the image have recovered fully between pulses and thus have the shortest T$_1$. However, if motion has occurred, as in the case of arterial blood, little NMR signal is received by the scanner and would therefore appear as a black area on the NMR image (Fig. 6.12). A full discussion of the measurement of T$_2$ by adjusting interpulse interval and T rep RF pulses and the effect of the T$_2$ component on NMR images is somewhat outside the scope of an introductory text; however, it is important to remember that T$_2$ can improve lesion detection (Fig. 6.13) and proton precessional coherence and thus T$_2$ transverse magnetization M$_{xy}$ is lost by two processes: (a) due to the external field nonuniformity, which in clinical scanning is on the order of 1 part in 10^4 or so, and (b) due to local spin-spin resonance flipping and nonuniformities in the local magnetic field within the tissue. The T$_2$ relaxation time is important when utilizing the spin-echo technique in NMR imaging, but unlike the FID in saturation recovery or inversion recovery where T$_2$ has little effect on T$_1$, the length of T$_1$ can have a significant effect on the intensity of the spin-echo. If the rep rate is shortened so that net tissue magnetization M$_z$ is not completely reestablished, then the z-oriented magnetization factor at the beginning of the spin-echo sequence (90° RF$_x$) will start out weaker, and the resultant M$_{xy}$ and thus the spin-echo will be weaker as well. In other words, a long T$_1$ will tend to decrease the intensity of the spin-echo signal.

For the purposes of this book, it is sufficient to restate that long T$_2$s provide more intense signals than short T$_2$ tissues and that lengthening the interpulse interval will often tend to magnify these differences (Fig. 6.9). As a further generalization, the width of the spin-

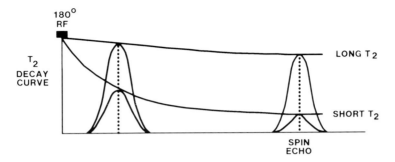

FIG. 6.9. In imaging sequences using the spin-echo technique, following the 180° RF pulse, although the T_2 of all tissues will decrease, those with a longer T_2 will demonstrate a stronger NMR signal as compared with a tissue with a shorter T_2 resulting in improved contrast enhancement and tissue lesion detectability. (See Figs. 6.3 to 6.5.)

echo is usually related directly to external field inhomogeneities, whereas the loss of height from the original fixed induction decay is mostly due to local magnetic fields in the tissue.

SPATIAL ENCODING

The NMR principles discussed so far are used in NMR spectroscopy, but the output is still in the form of spectroscopic squiggles. The question is, just how are we going to get a medical image out of all this?

The problem at this point is to find some way to locate in space from where the NMR signal is coming. If that were possible, then within the scanning area, we could assign a given signal back to a certain location and from there, reconstruct a cross-sectional image, as in the CT analogy. What is needed is some sort of spatial encoding of the NMR signal. It is probably easiest to understand how this is done if we again borrow a little bit more from our sonic analogy.

You are probably more familiar with spatially coded information than you are aware. For example, if we were to strike the note E from an octave on the piano, you could with some certainty say that the key that produced that tone was toward the left side of the octave. Essentially, you have used your knowledge of the general layout of a piano keyboard and coordinated that with the auditory cue. When the piano is tuned, lower tension (field strength) is placed on those strings that produce the lower notes, and progressively higher tension (field strength) is applied to those strings that produce the higher notes; by convention the gradient runs from left to right.

If we consider a piano player sitting at the keyboard, he essentially has learned to play the piano by memorizing which notes are associated with the keys and training his muscles to know how to find the appropriate key without looking or with few visual cues. Any remote listener with a similar knowledge of the keyboard could tell which key had been depressed simply by listening to the note struck by the piano player, even if he (the listener) were circling in a satellite in outer space far away from the piano. A listener with a good ear could specifically determine which key had been struck when we depressed the E key.

By using two piano keyboards (labeled x and y) oriented perpendicular to each other, we could then very accurately locate a point within a square determined by the two piano keyboards by listening to a two-note sequence. For example, if the note E were struck on the first piano, it would indicate third from the left (3_x), as in the previous example, and if a second note E were struck indicating a position third from the left (3_y) on the other piano keyboard, by extending the position of these two notes across the square at the intersection of those two projections, we would define a precise point in two-dimensional space between the two keyboards (Fig. 6.10). Extending this analogy through the third dimension, we could also describe any point within a cube defined by three piano keyboards (x, y, and z) located perpendicular to each other by any three note sequence. By projecting the position of these three piano keys, we could very accurately locate a point in space and anyone hearing these three notes would know exactly which point was being indicated. In reality we do not have a little man running around inside of each human being knocking out three tone signals so that we can determine, for example, the proton density of the liver.

The principle of NMR incorporates the concept of exciting tissue with RF electromagnetic waves and "listening" with an antenna or RF coil for the resonance frequency of the nuclear species excited. To illustrate how the RF signal is processed, let us assume for the moment that we have an imaginary tissue that is composed of small TV receiver-transmitters instead of protons. The TV station WNMR broadcasts the programs "60 Minutes", "CHiPs," and "Flo" with the same radio frequency and beams the channel at the TV receiver-transmitters within the tissue. Each TV-set receiver-transmitter would pick up the programs and visually transmit all three programs to an off-site viewer. We, as the viewer, would know that we have three channel selections, A, B, and C, but since we were receiving

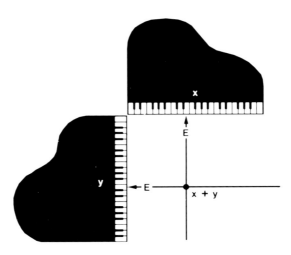

FIG. 6.10. Sound waves can be used to locate a given point in space. A remote listener hearing a two-note sequence and provided with the knowledge that two piano keyboards were at right angles to each other could correctly identify the intersection of the projection of the two lines (for example, E—tenth from the left x axis and E—tenth from the left y axis). Thus, the two-note sequence has spatially encoded information within it. A third piano keyboard along the z axis could similarly locate any point in three-dimensional space. In NMR imaging radio-frequency waves rather than sound waves can be manipulated to carry spatially encoded information. In the NMR scanner, however, gradient coils enable the examiner to select specifically the RF frequencies that correspond to certain positions in space.

all three programs on each channel, we would have no idea where the receiving antenna was within the tissue (Fig. 6.11).

However, if WNMR changed its programming policy and assigned a different signal for each program and we now equipped each receiving station with the appropriate UHF, VHF or short-wave antenna, only receiver A would receive "60 Minutes," only receiver B would pick up "CHiPs," and only receiver C would receive "Flo." Now by turning the dial on our channel selector, when we got "60 Minutes," we would know that it corresponded to receiver-transmitter A, and when we got "CHiPs," that would correspond to receiver-transmitter B, and when we received "Flo," we could assign that position to C and have some idea within the tissue where the receiver-transmitters were located (see Fig. 6.11).

In NMR imaging the principles are not very different from those described in the TV analogy. We are able to determine where a given proton is located in space by a technique that is very similar to changing the antenna to fit a certain TV channel (resonant fre-

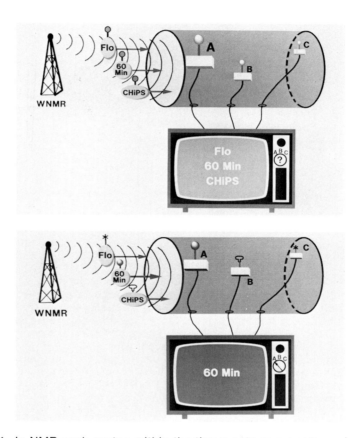

FIG. 6.11. In NMR each proton within the tissue acts as a small receiver-transmitter that absorbs and then retransmits the broadcast radio frequency pulse. If a TV station WNMR is broadcasting three programs ("Flo," "60 Minutes," and "CHiPs") on the same frequency, we should be unable to determine the position of receiver-transmitter antenna within a sample or tissue by turning the TV dial to the three receiver-transmitter to which we were connected. However, if each program was broadcast with a special frequency and each receiver-transmitter was equipped with a similarly matched antenna, then by turning the dial only the A channel would receive "60 Minutes," and we could identify the spatial position of that receiver-transmitter. In NMR imaging the selectivity of the *antenna* of the protons is established by applying a gradient magnetic field.

quency), and the method that allows us to perform this act in a functional sense without physically attaching a small separate antenna to every individual proton is to superimpose a magnetic gradient on the static magnetic field. As reviewed above, the frequency of magnetic resonance for a specific nuclear species is dependent on the strength of the magnetic field ($\omega = \gamma B$). This is specifically given by the

Larmor equation where the field-frequency relation for hydrogen is 42.58 MH_z/T. All forms of NMR imaging use some type of spatially encoded frequency discrimination to allow formation of the image. The major concept to bear in mind is that the stronger the magnetic field, the higher the precessional resonant frequency, and thus the higher the energy exchanged when flipping between low- and high-energy states. The potential for spatial encoding of a magnetic field is easily demonstrated when a deflected compass needle is noted to oscillate at its resonant frequency in the magnetic field of a bar magnet (Fig. 6.12). However, when the compass needle is advanced toward the magnet, one notices that the resonant frequency increases. The result is that the frequency of oscillation (new resonant frequency) increases, and it is the change in the strength of the magnetic field of the bar magnet that has produced this in the resonant frequency of the compass needle itself. Moving the compass needle into a higher magnetic field strength is equivalent in a sense to tightening the string on a piano to tune it to a note of higher frequency

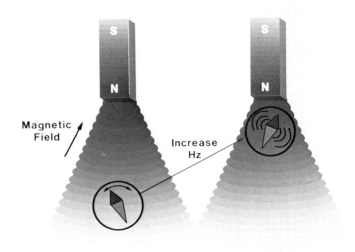

FIG. 6.12. The strength of the magnetic field will influence the natural frequency of vibration of a compass needle such that if the compass is moved closer to the magnet and into higher field strength, the frequency will increase. This predictable relationship between frequency and magnetic field strength is the mechanism in NMR scanning which, by knowing the field strength and measuring the frequency, a given position in space can be identified. In other words, the frequency has spatially encoded information.

or higher energy. Therefore, in a gradient magnetic field, we can assign a position in space by knowing the precessional frequency and the size of the magnetic field at that point.

We can represent the spatial encoding in NMR, as depicted in Fig. 6.13. The object is placed in a static magnetic field (B), and subsequently a gradient magnetic field is applied. Planes in the figure correspond to higher or lower positions on the gradient magnetic field. This results in correspondingly higher or lower resonant frequency, respectively, and these frequencies can be related back to the gradient magnetic field and the corresponding spatial location of the planes identified. Additional information is present in the signal because the amplitude of the resonant frequencies corresponds to the amount of material present at that location.

Following the same line of reasoning, we can localize any nucleus in three-dimensional space by placing a magnetic gradient on the x, y, and z axes in a similar fashion to the way we placed three piano keyboards on the x, y, and z axes to locate a point in space by a three-note combination. In this case we would have unique precessional frequencies, and knowing what frequency corresponded with a certain position in the magnetic gradient, we could then localize any desired point in space. It is important to keep in mind that although a magnetic gradient can be established in either the x, y, or z direction (through various manipulations of the gradient coils and

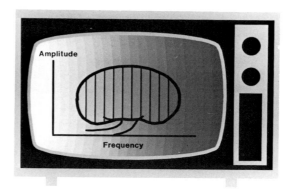

FIG. 6.13. In NMR scanning the radio-frequency signal has amplitude information that corresponds to the amount or the number of hydrogen nuclei present. The frequency of the RF signal can be used to locate the nuclei in space due to the fact that the frequency increases with increasing magnetic field strength. Thus, the signal, in this case from a conceptualized kidney, can be thought of as an amplitude vs frequency plot from which the general outline and character of the tissue can be determined.

technical modifications of the NMR imaging system), the static magnetic field by definition points along the z axis. It is the direction of the gradient rather than the direction of the static magnetic field that is important for spatial encoding.

GRADIENT IMAGING

In NMR a linear gradient magnetic field causes frequency to bear a relationship to position. The concept of utilizing a linear gradient in the magnetic field in conjunction with an image reconstruction technique, which had been previously used in conjunction with CT scanning, i.e., filtered back projection, was put forward by Lauterbur in his 1973 article in *Nature*. To reconstruct a three-dimensional image of the body, three such linear gradients are used, which are perpendicular to each other. Nevertheless, the general principle, as we have just reviewed, is to relate a specific frequency to a specific geometric location. The difference between the NMR imaging process and the spectroscopic process is that each point is located with a specific frequency by gradient coil in NMR imaging.

We shall discuss filtered back projection and other reconstruction imaging techniques in more detail in the next chapter. However, the methodology is somewhat analogous to the problem of trying to determine the configuration of an object placed inside a lamp shade and tracing its contours on the shade in several different places and subsequently projecting back to the intersection of all of these traced images to define the location and configuration of the object itself. In general, the more tracings that are made to try to define the configuration (the more angles of view or the more projections), the more accurate the final configuration is likely to be. The amplitude of radio waves used in NMR, as opposed to the light waves used in the lamp shade problem, correspond to the amount of material (hydrogen) located at a given location. In other words, the frequency indicates the spatial location, and the amplitude indicates the amount of material present.

SELECTIVE EXCITATION

Imaging Techniques

Previously, we have seen how it is possible to irradiate a tissue with a broad range of radio frequencies and with a magnetic field gradient to determine the position that a given nuclear receiver-transmitter has by its emitted characteristic resonant frequency. Since the resonant frequency of hydrogen and other nuclear species capable of nuclear magnetic resonance are known, it is also possible to use a single coherent frequency (as opposed to a broad band) to locate a thin plane of tissue for which the gradient magnetic field and frequency match.

In order to grasp this concept, it may be useful to return to the WNMR transmitter. If WNMR transmits only a one-frequency signal (60″) and similarly tuned receiver-transmitters are aligned in planes, then only a thin plane of the appropriate "tuned" receiver-transmitter antenna will be excited, and our TV receiver will find that 60″ signals are only transmitted from a very thinly defined plane. In NMR imaging we would achieve this selectivity of proton receiver-transmitters by applying the gradient magnetic field. If we retain the information from the original plane of excitation and now move WNMR perpendicular to the tissue, and again irradiate the tissue with a different frequency signal, a new plane perpendicular to the first will be the only one absorbing the signal and again subsequently rebroadcasting (transmitting) to our TV receiver on the other side. An observer would then be in a position to define either one of the two planes or define the single receiver-transmitter by the intersection of three planes. In NMR imaging this rearrangement of the receiver-transmitter antenna would be achieved by alternately applying perpendicular gradient magnetic fields. Following a similar procedure for three-dimensional imaging, we could also define a third plane perpendicular to the first two and find the single voxel (volume of tissue) defined by the receiver-transmitter at the exact center of the intersection of the three planes.

By selective excitation in NMR, we can excite only those nuclei (protons) in a thin slice of the body or those in a single line or a single voxel. In NMR this is generally accomplished by applying one gradient during excitation and then applying a second or third gradient perpendicular to it during the readout. In actual practice, the excitation RF pulse is a broadcast of many frequencies, and in effect each proton becomes a small transmitter. The information contained has spatial encoding in the frequency of each signal, and signals from many protons are transmitted at once. The RF signal also has information about the number of proton transmitters and the character of the tissue obtained in the amplitude or strength of the energy. In

NMR imaging selective excitation is accomplished by manipulating the net magnetization vector with the appropriate RF pulse (90° RF_x and 180° RF_x) to define the plane or line or point of interest.

You will recall from Chapter 5 that by using an RF pulse for the appropriate duration and along the appropriate axis, we can actually tip net tissue magnetization through any number of desired degrees of rotation. Essentially, three-dimensional spatial encoding in magnetic resonance combines the gradient magnetic field with various degrees of RF pulse rotation to isolate planes, lines, and points of tissue with uniquely oriented magnetic dipoles and net magnetization. If, for example, a given RF pulse tips the net magnetization vector M 90° (90° RF_x), then a pulse with twice the strength or twice the duration will cause a further displacement of M so that it lies along the $-z$ axis or a 180° shift (180° RF_x) (see Fig. 5.12).

By combining the techniques of inversion recovery and gradient manipulation, three-dimensional spatial information can be determined as follows: after a 180° pulse, the net tissue magnetization is directed along the $-z$ axis in all volume elements in the tissue (Fig. 6.14). After a period τ, a 90° RF_x pulse is applied with a z gradient such that only those volume elements in a plane parallel to the xy plane are rotated 90° (Fig. 6.15). As transverse relaxation occurs within the excited 90° RF_x plane, additional x and y gradients are applied to provide spatial information for points within the plane. In volume elements outside the excited plane, the magnetization continues to recover along the z axis.

One additional technique used in NMR imaging that is likely to become more important as experience with this technology progresses is the spin-echo technique. The spin-echo is a magnetic resonance signal that returns after the last excitation pulse. The amplitude of the spin-echo indicates the number of protons involved and how well they remain in phase (coherent). The frequency of the spin-echo indicates the strength of the local magnetic field, which is determined by gradient manipulations.

To begin spatial encoding with the spin-echo technique, a magnetic gradient is applied along the y axis (Fig. 6.16). The sample is then exposed to a 90° pulse from an RF coil along the x axis (90° RF_x). Only part of the sample—the stimulated or excited volume—at a specific magnetic field strength will resonate with the exact frequency of the 90° pulse. The magnetization M of the excited volume that was pointing along the z axis is now rotated 90° so that it points along the

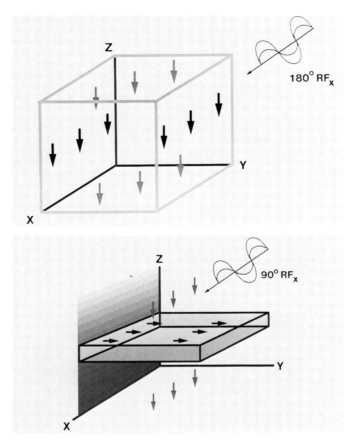

FIGS. 6.14 and 6.15. The inversion-recovery imaging sequence can be used to provide spatially encoded information. In this sequence a 180° RF$_x$ pulse inverts the protons in the sample (*top*), and subsequently (*bottom*) a gradient is applied along the z axis and a 90° RF$_x$ is pulsed into the tissue at a frequency that is specific for one of the frequency bands identified by the gradient along the z axis. Thus, only those protons in the plane defined by the specific magnetic gradient and matching the frequency of the RF pulse will be shifted 90° along the y axis. Protons outside this plane will continue to be inverted and slowly relax along the z axis. Thus, the NMR signal obtained will be specific for only the plane defined. A gradient perpendicular to this plane would similarly define a line within that plane, and a plane gradient perpendicular to this could define any voxel desired and an image reconstructed on a basis of this selective information.

y axis (see Fig. 6.9). As with inversion recovery, those protons outside the excited volume (i.e., outside the plane parallel to the xz axis remain parallel to the z axis). At this point, a magnetic gradient along the z axis is applied, and a 180° RF$_x$ pulse is used to irradiate the

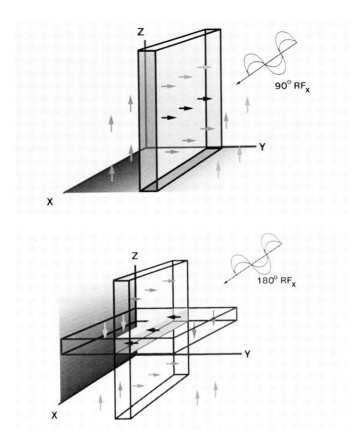

FIGS. 6.16 and 6.17. The spin-echo technique can also be used to spatially encode NMR signal information. In this sequence a gradient is applied along the y axis (*top*) and a 90° RF$_x$ pulse transmitted to the sample. Again, only those protons precessing at the resonant frequency defined by the gradient will respond to the 90° shift and orient along the y axis. Subsequently, the xy gradient is turned off, and a gradient along the z axis is applied. The tissue is irradiated with an 180° RF$_x$ pulse in this second situation (*bottom*). Again, only those protons in the plane defined by the specific, matching RF frequency and gradient will shift 180°. This results in inversion of the previously nonexcited nuclei, but those nuclei excited during the 90° RF pulse will now point in the −y direction, thus defining a line. A similar gradient perpendicular to these two can then define a voxel. In practice, these gradients are often applied and shifted during both the irradiation and readout phases, but in any event, any voxel in space can be defined using these techniques and the image reconstructed from these individually coded voxels.

tissue (Fig. 6.17). The z gradient again selects only that plane that will respond to the 180° RF_x pulse, which is a plane parallel to the plane of xy. Again, the protons that are outside of the two excited planes remain pointing along the z axis. Only those protons at the intersection of the two excited planes will be pointing in the $-y$ direction and therefore have a uniquely encoded net magnetization or NMR signal. (Protons in the xy plane volume excited by the 180° RF_x pulse generally point in the $-z$ direction.)

Chapter 7

Nuclear Magnetic Resonance Image Reconstruction Techniques

In the preceding chapters, we have been developing the concept that one of the most exciting aspects of NMR is its capability to produce medical images based on four separate characteristics of tissue. As in CT, a cross-sectional NMR image can be produced, i.e., an NMR image can resolve organ structure on the basis of depth. However, one NMR image can be constructed based on the proton density of the tissue; another can be created representing the T_1 relaxation time distribution of the same section; in a similar fashion, a third image of the section can be created representing T_2 relaxation time distribution; and another NMR image sensitive to flow can be reconstructed. The NMR signal from anything that is rapidly moving and taken out of the imaging plan will not be recorded by the RF receiver. Thus, little NMR signal will be obtained from those rapidly flowing structures such as the aorta, whereas slower flow from thrombosis or turbulence from an atherosclerotic plaque will have an increased NMR signal. Thus, an image can be created that reflects movement or flow within the cross section. Although some NMR imaging equipment is capable of producing calculated T_1 and T_2 images, in actual practice, most NMR images today represent an amalgamation of the four parameters, which have been blended to best illustrate the anatomy or pathology with which the radiologist and clinician are concerned.

As discussed in Chapter 6, a way of categorizing imaging techniques is according to the dimension of the excited volume. Assuming the total imaging volume to be divided into n_x, n_y, and n_z volume elements (voxels) along the three spatial coordinates, then n_x, n_y, n_z signal elements are required to reconstruct the images within this volume. In the simplest imaging experiment the signal of each voxel is acquired independently. This method therefore, has been termed the sequential point or null point method. Sequential line and sequential plane methods are also used. In three-dimensional imaging, the signals of all voxels are observed at the same time. Currently, sequential point and line methods have largely been abandoned because signals are gathered from a relatively small number of nuclei. However, planar and volume imaging methods are computationally more demanding. Among the generally adopted planar and volume imaging techniques, two methods have evolved: multiple angle projection-reconstruction techniques and spin-warp imaging.

Briefly, multiple angle projection reconstruction was first proposed by Lauterbur and closely resembles X-ray CT reconstruction. It consists of rotating a gradient in small angular displacements to produce, for each angle increment, a projection or view. The advantage of the multiple angle projection-reconstruction technique is its relative simplicity and the use of well-established (from X-ray CT) algorithms for image reconstruction. However, in NMR scanning it has the disadvantage of being sensitive to motion artifacts and field inhomogeneity.

Phase encoding and spin-warp imaging experiments use a succession of three time periods and magnetic gradients to create a cross-sectional image representing a plane, whose pixels are characterized by x and y coordinants. During the first RF pulse, one of two perpendicular gradients, G_x, is active. This gradient is turned off after t_x seconds and gradient G_y is activated, during which time (t_y) the FID is collected. During the two periods, the magnetization precesses at the frequencies determined by the strength of the magnetic field.

The frequency ω_y determines the location of the resonating spins with respect to y, but the accumulated phase angle of the precessing protons is spatially related to the x coordinate, since the magnetization for each location x is not only characterized by a unique frequency but also has a unique phase angle associated with it. The transverse magnetization vectors, when plotted against the y coordinate, are twisted in a spiral fashion comparable in appearance to the steps of circular stairway except that their lengths are related to the proton density at their respective locations. The image is obtained by collecting n FIDs. The resulting n × n data matrix is then Fourier transformed with each data point directly providing a specific voxel value. This method thus obviates the need for reconstruction techniques.

Spin warp imaging, first proposed by Edelstein et al., creates the phase twist by varying the gradient during the first RF pulse and holding t_x constant, which provides a similar accumulated phase angle related to the x axis. The main advantage of spin warp over other imaging techniques is the fact that it is relatively tolerant to static magnetic field inhomogeneities. These inhomogeneities do affect signal phase, however, the effect is the same in each of the FIDs and is eliminated at the end of processing. A further benefit of the spin warp method is its relative insensitivity to irregular motion such as breathing, or peristaltic patient motion. Both projection-reconstruction and 2D Fourier imaging can be extended to a third dimension. In the latter method, this is accomplished by applying x and z gradients (G_x and G_z) during the excitation period. During the readout period, a gradient G_y is turned on. In this case, the accumulated phase angle at the starting time of data acquisition is a function of both coordinants x and z. In 3D spin warp the gradients G_x and G_z are incremented in steps. From such scans, transverse, sagittal coronal and off-angle images across any point within the imaged volume can rapidly be displayed.

The three reconstruction methods used in producing images from NMR signals that are in common use today are: zeugmatography, two-dimensional Fourier transform (2DFT), and three-dimensional Fourier transform (3DFT). Each of these methods will be discussed in this chapter.

BACK PROJECTION ZEUGMATOGRAPHY

Zeugmatography as related to NMR imaging was originally described by Lauterber in 1973 and, as previously mentioned in Chapter 2, implies the yoking together of the magnetic fields and of nuclear magnetic resonance and electromagnetic waves in the radio-frequency range. Essentially, the NMR information is utilized to produce a "picture" of the internal structure of the human body or, for that matter, any tissue or structure having magnetic nuclei within it.

The techniques involve the obtaining of many projections and is similar to the problem faced by the investigator who has been given the task of determining what, if any, structures have been placed in a room that is surrounded on all four sides by a sheet over which he cannot see. The only tools he is given to solve the problem are a light bulb inside the room that he can move by a remote control and a piece of chalk. His approach in solving this problem is a simplified version of that which is utilized in CT and zeugmatography imaging. The investigator walks around the perimeter of the room always keeping the light bulb against the far wall perpendicular to him and stopping at various points to trace the shadow cast by the objects in the room on the sheet. After outlining all the silhouettes, the investigator draws perpendicular lines from each of the shadows cast on the sheet and projects them back to their point of intersection in the room. From these "back projections," he constructs his best estimate of the position and configuration of the objects in the room. Of course, if he takes the time to take more projections, he can come closer to the true configuration and placement of the objects in the room, and this same principle is equally true of magnetic resonance and CT reconstruction techniques, i.e., the more angles of view one obtains, the more accurate the image will be.

In NMR back projection imaging as well as in back projection imaging in CT, the reconstruction problem is very similar except that computers do the work of reconstruction. The technique involves the obtaining of many projections, and then after some computer filtering to eliminate background noise, and other imaging process techniques back projecting the data, i.e., proton density data, the image can be obtained.

The first step in this process is to place the object or area of interest within the aperture of the circular magnet of the NMR scanner. A central portion of this aperture is arbitrarily divided up into a grid-like matrix of rectangular cells called *voxels,* which have a finite depth usually determined by the slice thickness elected for the scanning procedure (i.e., voxel = volume element) and a square arbitrarily defined end-surface called the *pixel* (i.e., pixel = picture element). Picture elements are so-called because they represent in two-dimensional imaging the data obtained from the volume of tissue scanned, and since most of the scans are viewed on a TV picture tube [cathode-ray (CRT) tube], the pixel is usually the basic element used on most NMR or CT scanner systems.

After the grid-like matrix has been established, multiple projections of a patient can be made by changing the direction of the gradient in the x, y, and z planes and back projecting these data to form an image of the objects in cross section, as illustrated in Fig. 7.1. As mentioned previously, the data used to reconstruct the image can be either proton density or T_1 or T_2 relaxation time, or a combination of all three of these parameters. In any event, after many projections are obtained, the computer assigns to each volume element the mean value for the volume of tissue scanned in that element, and this value is then assigned to the pixel for viewing on the CRT.

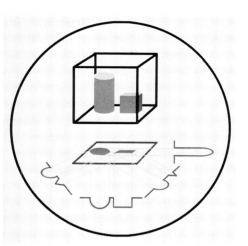

FIG. 7.1. In the filtered back projection method of image reconstruction which is the method used in X-ray CT scanning, multiple projections of the desired volume are obtained. The amplitude of the NMR signal is used to assign the amount or number of nuclei present, and the frequency of the signal is used to assign the spatial location. Multiple projections or angles of view are obtained by back projecting these multiple views. The objects contained within the scanning area can be resolved. In practice, in order to image a matrix of N × N pixels N angles of view with N points (detectors) per view are required.

Of course, the signal obtained is not electromagnetic wave information in the form of visible light, as in the problem presented above, but rather electromagnetic wave information in the form of radio waves with the amount of proton density encoded in the amplitude of the signal and the spacial localization encoded in the frequency of the signal. Conversion between the two components of the signal— time and frequency—is accomplished by the Fourier transformation, which was discussed in Chapter 5.

TWO- AND THREE-DIMENSIONAL IMAGING

We have seen previously how it is possible to encode spatial information by using a magnetic gradient because of the dependency of resonant frequency on regional magnetic field strength. Thus, knowing a given frequency, we are able to assign a position in space to the nuclei emitting that frequency. It is also possible to encode spatial information by making the position in the precessional rotation about the static magnetic field correspond to spatial information.

One way to approach this problem is to put yourself in the position of a baseball coach who needs a fast player to steal bases. The problem is to keep track, in some way, of five baseball players (A to E) who are trying out for the team. The coach decides to record player performance on baseball diamond drawings. However, the circumstances arose in which each successive batter had a base hit, resulting in A, B, and C being on third, second, and first base, respectively. Subsequently, batter D also hit a single advancing A to home for the first run but using the picture of the diamond for a record, it is difficult to determine if A or E has just scored. An alternative way of keeping track of the players' base running ability is to let each player's position be represented by his progress around the four bases of the diamond. This eliminates the confusion as to whether A or E is up to bat or has just scored the first run. In this method of keeping track of the players, E is assigned the initial starting position O, D one-quarter, C one-half, B three-quarters, and A one, indicating their progression around the bases (Fig. 7.2). It might also be possible to assign the baseball players a position on a sine wave with a recurring pattern to represent their respective positions. As more runs are made, the players could be advanced through successive sine wave cycles (see Fig. 7.2).

TWO- AND THREE-DIMENSIONAL FOURIER TRANSFORM

Fourier transform reconstruction is similar to phase encoding baseball players. In NMR imaging using the two-dimensional Fourier transform (2DFT) reonstruction methodology, a set of voxels in an

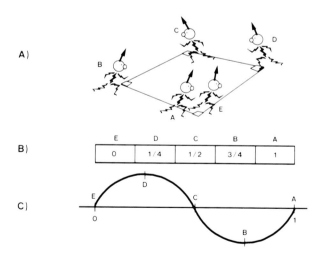

FIG. 7.2. Four baseball players have identical speed, or their frequency in rounding the bases is identical; keeping track of their base running ability by merely monitoring their speed is not satisfactory. One way of approaching this situation would be to assign a base running phase to each player. In this case, as the base runners come up to home plate and begin their cycle around the diamond, runner A who has just completed one cycle can be differentiated from runner E who has yet to begin. Each successive player can then be assigned a value depending on his position in the cycle, and this similarly can be represented by a cycling sine wave as illustrated in **C.**

xy plane is defined with a z gradient. A second gradient applied along the x axis again permits positions along the x axis to be frequency encoded, and a row of voxels along the y axis can be defined. Up to this time, we have applied no gradient along the y axis and therefore, the precessional frequencies are equal along the y axis. In addition, the precessing magnetization vectors of these tissue voxels remain in phase. In order to assign a unique characteristic to each voxel so that the NMR signal could be immediately assigned to any given voxel in three-dimensional space (thus precluding the necessity for filtered back projection), a special magnetic gradient could be added along the y axis specifically to provide phase shifts in the precessing nuclei (Fig. 7.3). The y gradient is applied so that magnetization of the voxel in the strongest field (A) is one cycle ahead of that in the weakest field (E) when the gradient is turned off, at which point this row of voxels would again experience the static magnetic field along the z axis and continue to precess at the same frequency; yet, they are out of phase in a predictable way with each other. We can record these phase shifts by using a sine wave representation similar to the methodology used to keep track of baseball players in spring practice (see Fig. 7.3). Each shift in phase would encode spatial information along the y axis. Imaging requires a sequence of many phases since the sum of voxels of different phases is all that can be resolved.

By expanding the amount of tissue irradiated and using a combi-

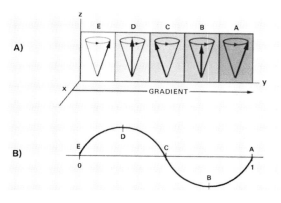

FIG. 7.3. In 3-D Fourier reconstruction, phase encoding the NMR signal is similar to phase encoding the basebll players in Fig. 7.2. For example, a gradient is applied prior to RF tissue irradiation so that each nucleus is precessing at a slightly different but defined rate. The gradient is then switched off and the imaging sequence begins, such that the defined voxels are precessing at the same precessional frequency, but they are out of phase with each other in a defined way. Thus, although the precessional frequency for each voxel is identical, the phase shift represents a specific spatial signature, and this information can be used to reconstruct the image. Fig. 6.1 was reconstructed by a 3-D Fourier transformation method.

nation of phase and frequency encoding around two axes instead of just the y axis, large volumes of tissue can be encoded with spatial information. The advantage in this regard is that since each voxel has a unique value directly assigned to it, rather than being assigned a value from filtered back projection, sagittal, coronal, or oblique reconstructions can be performed very quickly once the data are obtained without having to completely rescan with a sagittal or coronal or oblique orientation. The speed with which these reconstructions can be performed may be a big advantage in magnetic resonance imaging.

Both zeugmatography and three-dimensional Fourier transform (3DFT) are whole volume irradiation techniques. The fundamental difference between the two techniques is that in zeugmatography imaging the entire object is projected onto a line, and the direction of the line projection is rotated in three dimensions around the object being scanned, i.e., many angles of view or projections of view are obtained. In 3DFT imaging the object is always projected onto the same line, and spatial encoding in the two directions perpendicular to the line of projection is accomplished by phase encoding the magnetic moments in a predictable way in these two directions.

Chapter 8

Nuclear Magnetic Resonance Imaging— History, State of the Art, and Future Potential

HISTORICAL PERSPECTIVE

The principles of magnetic resonance were originally developed at Stanford by Block for liquids and at Harvard by Purcell for solids in 1946. They subsequently received the Nobel Prize for their observations in 1952. In 1951 Gabillard first noted that spatial localization was potentially possible with magnetic resonance. The current generation of imaging techniques received most of their impetus from the publication in *Nature* by Lauterbur in 1973 regarding a spatial coding and back projection reconstruction technique in magnetic resonance which he termed *zeugmatography*. In 1975 EMI began prototype development of a commercial magnetic resonance scanner, and subsequently from 1980 to 1983 pilot clinical trials (FONAR, GEC Technicare, Nottingham, Aberdeen, and Diasonics) were underway. Although there was a limited number of magnetic resonance scanners capable of human imaging in the initial period, the enthusiasm for the potential of NMR was an indication of the unique qualities that this modality possesses.

As discussed previously, the NMR signal is based on a very complex set of tissue parameters, including hydrogen density, two separate relaxation times, T_1 and T_2, and since it takes a finite time to register the signal emitted by the excited hydrogen nuclei, there is no NMR signal recorded by the RF signal from fast-moving nuclei. In other words, the technique is very sensitive to flow. By using these four parameters for ^1H, a wealth of clinical information is potentially available from NMR studies. This is in contrast to the signal obtained from transmission X-ray computed tomography (CT), for example, where the information is largely based on a physical characteristic—tissue electron density. The difference is comparable to being able to resolve a blood protein on the one hand with only a single dimension electrophoretic gel diffusion and on the other being able to separate proteins with a three-dimensional or cubic gel with two electrophoretic gradients plus a chemical gradient.

Future Potential of Magnetic Resonance Imaging in Medicine

The capability of being able to localize anatomically the information from magnetic resonance spectroscopy is a very powerful concept. If the promise is ever fulfilled, it could be like a real time organ specific image of biomolecular events. The NMR signal, as reviewed, is potentially at least four times as rich as the CT signal. But the NMR signal is even more sophisticated than this. By using specialized magnetic resonance techniques, there are many other nuclear species that have magnetic moments and are potentially imageable in the body.

NUCLEAR MAGNETIC RESONANCE IMAGING WITH OTHER NUCLEAR SPECIES

To be potentially capable of being imaged by NMR, nuclei should be biologically prevalent and also magnetic. For example, although ^{12}C is prevalent within the body, it is not magnetic. The isotope ^{13}C

is magnetic and potentially useful as a magnetic resonance agent, but its biological abundance is only approximately 1%. Thus, the combination of concentration, natural abundance, and the intrinsic relative NMR signal strength gives the overall NMR signal sensitivity. In Table 8.1 the nuclei of greatest interest in NMR imaging in medicine are listed in order of their decreasing NMR sensitivity.

Sodium-23 has actually been used to produce a cross-sectional NMR images, and the preliminary results are extremely encouraging. Current studies being conducted at Harvard Medical School and elsewhere have produced gated images of isolated perfused hearts bathed in a perfusate with high sodium concentration. Similar studies have been conducted *in vivo* in the cat. These studies are encouraging because most of the body sodium is outside of the cell, and when the cell membrane is damaged, sodium is allowed to flood the intracellular compartments. Observing this phenomenon may indicate areas of ischemic or infarcted tissue in the brain, heart, or other body organs. One of the most exciting concepts in NMR imaging, however, is the potential to perform chemical shift imaging and image triggered spectroscopy.

IMAGING SPECTROSCOPY

Chemical Shift Imaging

We have dealt with the nucleus (^{1}H) as essentially having a single resonant frequency dictated by the magnetic field $\omega = \gamma B$. However, in biological samples containing molecules, the magnetic field that is experienced by a nucleus is modified by the surrounding electrons or the regional molecular environment. These bonding electrons introduce a factor called the *chemical shielding factor* and the true resonant frequency equation for a nuclear species is given by the

TABLE 8.1. *Properties of nuclei of interest in medicine*

Nucleus	Spin	MHz/T
^{1}H	1/2	42.6
^{2}H	1	6.5
^{13}C	1/2	16.7
^{14}N	1	3.1
^{15}N	$-1/2$	9.3
^{17}O	$-5/2$	5.8
^{19}F	1/2	40.1
^{23}Na	3/2	11.3
^{31}p	1/2	17.2

formula $\omega = \gamma B \times (1 - \sigma)$. This electron screening (or reduction in the magnetic field experienced by the nucleus) as it is called results in nuclei from different chemical (electromagnetic) environments having slightly different resonant frequencies, which produce a spectrum of Lorentzian lines (very narrow bandwidths of a few hertz in width), reflecting the same nuclear species with variable electron screening. The areas under these lines are proportional to the relative concentrations of the corresponding nuclei and the width is related to T_2.

In 1950 it was discovered that not all nuclei of the same type have identical resonance frequency at a given field strength. With this discovery, whole new areas of NMR applications were established. The essential result of the large number of studies conducted to date, however, is that we can now study *in vivo* chemistry. At this point only small volumes of tissue can be analyzed by NMR chemistry; however, when this information is superimposed on a hydrogen map or hydrogen density scan and associated with anatomical localization within the body, this methodology can be extremely powerful. The first reported example of this chemical shift effect was for nitrogen (^{14}N) where two signals were observed from a solution of ammonium nitrate (NH_4NO_3); one signal was detected from each nitrogen atom. The differences in resonant frequency are small (on the order of 5 to 30 parts per million) and are termed *chemical shifts*. These separations are proportional to the applied magnetic field and hence are more easily seen in higher field magnets. Because the chemical shifts are so small, the magnetic field must be very homogeneous ($>1/10^6$) or the chemical shift will be obscured by the noise background. Narrow resonance lines are generally only found for small molecules in solution as opposed to solid state NMR or NMR of solids.

NMR spectra also exhibit spin-spin coupling (which should not be confused with spin-spin relaxation or T2)—in addition to the chemical shift—which is a manifestation of nuclear/nuclear interactions that are transmitted via the binding electrons. In other words, if a magnetic nucleus (say the γ phosphorous in ATP is connected via one or two chemical bonds to another chemically distinct nucleus (i.e., the β phosphorous of ATP in Fig. 8.1), then the first nucleus can sense (be exposed to different magnetic fields) the two resonance states of the β phosphorus and vice versa. Hence, their resonant peaks are split into doublet, as illustrated in Fig. 8.1. As in proton imaging, the T_1 (spin-lattice) and the T_2 (spin-spin) relaxation times can be used to characterize the resonance lines. These relaxation times are a func-

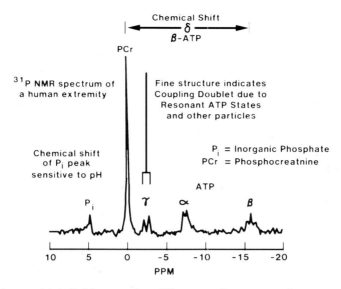

FIG. 8.1. At very high field strengths, differences in resonant frequency between identical nuclei can be detected, as illustrated in this spectroscopy experiment of the phosphorus from a human extremity. The α, γ, and β phosphorus peaks in ATP, for example, can be detected from each other due to their differing regional chemical (and therefore magnetic) environment. In addition, the double-spiked peak of the γ phosphorus can be detected, and this shift in the spectrum is due to the spin-spin coupling between the γ phosphorus and the resonant states of other phosphorus atoms in the ATP molecule. In other words, the status of the adjacent phosphorus resonant states influences the magnetic environment of the γ phosphorus. This type of information may be valuable when used in conjunction with NMR imaging.

tion of the motion of the molecule and describe the time response of a nucleus to a perturbation that disturbs the equilibrium distribution of the nuclei. As Fig. 8.1 indicates, changes in inorganic phosphorus (Pi) reflect changes in local chemical pH, and the phosphocreatine (PCr) and three phosphorus molecules of ATP give a good deal of information about the relative metabolic activity of the tissue. The information in these studies is given in relative (usually referenced to a PCr standard) values of parts per million to eliminate the effect of variable field strengths from one experiment to another.

Surface Coils and Topical Magnetic Resonance

First generation NMR imaging magnets had field homogeneities of a few parts in 10^4 or 10^5; therefore, they did not resolve these small chemical shift effects. However, field homogeneities of magnets at

1.5T and above do allow chemical shift imaging. Two techniques that are used to allow high resolution spectra to be obtained are the combined use of surface coils and topical magnetic resonance (TMR). The surface coils act by actually magnetizing a portion of the tissue below the surface to which they are applied, whereas the TMR methodology reforms the static magnetic field. With these techniques it is possible to obtain high-quality spectra from known localized volumes within a patient or animal. Chemical effects are important to *in vivo* biochemistry and chemical research. It is becoming possible to measure, in a totally noninvasive way, parameters such as intracellular pH and metabolic concentrations and to perform tracer studies without the use of radionuclei or ionizing radiation.

A flat surface coil will, under normal circumstances, excite and detect signals from an approximately disc-shaped region in front of the coil. The thickness and radius of this disc are approximately equal to the radius of the coil, although the excited field increases the deeper one goes from the skin surface. That is, the width of the sensitive volume increases with penetration. This drawback is compensated for by combining the surface coil with TMR techniques.

An additional set of profiling coils is placed inside the bore of a superconducting magnet that modifies the static magnetic field so that, within the sensitive volume selected, the magnetic field is uniform and, outside this volume, the magnetic field changes rapidly. Within the sensitive volume, the magnetic field inhomogeneities are less than the typical chemical shift linewidths and high resolution spectra can be acquired from that part of the sample that lies within this roughly spherical volume. Immediately adjacent to the central volume is a region where the magnetic field is changing very rapidly with position. Inhomogeneously broadened spectra will be acquired from this region since the range of signal frequencies will still lie within the bandwidth of the spectrometer receiver. In all other regions of the sample, the spectral lines will be broadened and shifted so much that the signal frequencies will lie outside the receiver bandwidth and will not be detected.

The medical applications of chemical shift imaging depend on the technological capability of providing homogeneous fields (1 in 10^6 or better) with a solenoid (cylindrical volume) configuration, so that patients can be placed within the scanners. One technique, which has been used to obtain three-dimensional spatial information with surface coils, entails placing the object to be scanned inside two opposing surface coils and the respective internal magnetic fields profiled with topical magnetic resonance technique. The profiling is done such that the fields covered a small section of the object. Then either by rotating the opposing surface coils or by rotating the object to be scanned, the entire internal volume is studied, and with careful profiling and rotating, a fairly accurate impression of the spatial configuration of the internal structures is obtained.

Electron Paramagnetic Resonance

Previously in this text we have considered the mechanism by which spinning particles can interact with the beam of electromagnetic radiation (RF). If the beam has the same frequency as that of the precessing particle, it can interact coherently with the particle, and energy can be exchanged. This is the phenomenon of resonance, and we have heretofore considered this interaction with nuclear species and referred to it as NMR. If the appropriate radiation (microwave) is broadcast into the tissues, however, unpaired electrons are also capable of coherently absorbing the energy. The magnetic fields required to record this interaction must be very homogeneous but usually of lower field strength, and this phenomenon is referred to as electron paramagnetic resonance (EPR) or, sometimes, electron spin resonance (ESR). ESR spectroscopy, or recording information from unpaired electrons in a given sample, is a well-established technology and it may well be possible at some point to spatially encode this information and perform ESR imaging, which would add a further dimension to the potential applications of chemical shift imaging in magnetic resonance.

^{1}H and Isotope Imaging

Although ^{1}H has virtually a 100% natural abundance and should give the largest NMR signal, the very strong water signal obtained from biological samples, coupled with the narrow spread of chemical shifts (very few parts per million), generally makes it difficult to study molecularly bound ^{1}H; nevertheless, chemical shifts of molecularly bound hydrogen have been studied and a typical spectrum from human extremities has demonstrated that the larger signals are primarily from H_2O in the muscle but that some of the acyl chains of triglyceride stored in fat can also be observed. A one pixel chemical shift image between water or fat protons was first demonstrated by GE at 1.5T.

^{31}P

In 1974 it was shown that ^{31}P spectra could be obtained from intact muscle. The NMR signals were identified as originating from the major phosphate metabolites in the cell, e.g., adenosine triphosphate (ATP), phosphocreatine (PCr), and inorganic phosphate (Pi). The presence of adenosine diphosphate (ADP) is generally masked, due to its low concentration and overlap with the ATP spectral lines.

The ^{31}P NMR spectra can provide detailed information about biochemical processes. For example, the relative concentrations of the metabolites can be measured from the area of the respective resonance lines and the position of the ATP lines indicates that the ATP is complexed to Mg^{2+} ions. In addition, intracellular pH can be measured since the chemical shift of the Pi line is very sensitive to pH in the biological range.

The localized ^{31}P spectra produced by TMR make it possible to identify and study the metabolism of specific tissues within the body. Since different classes of healthy tissue have characteristic amounts of the various phosphate metabolites, they will exhibit different characteristic spectra. For example, the primary fuel for skeletal muscle contraction is provided by the breakdown of ATP into ADP and Pi. The ATP level is replenished by PCr. PCr is, therefore, the energy reservoir of the muscle and, as might be expected, is stored at a high concentration in the healthy muscle, as is shown for the human arm in Fig. 8.1. In contrast, an organ such as the liver would not be expected to store PCr, and a low level of PCr should be seen in a liver spectrum. Diseased tissues have spectra that are distinct from healthy tissues.

^{31}P NMR is thus a powerful tool for studying metabolic pathways and energy conversion processes. Topical magnetic resonance enables *in vivo* measurements to be carried out in specific organs. Currently, the major applications of *in vivo* NMR chemical analysis concern phosphate metabolism. One of the potential medical adaptations of this capability is in detecting the differences in converting ADP to ATP under aerobic conditions with the production of carbon dioxide and water or anaerobic conditions with the production of lactic acid and thus cellular acidity. The latter pathway is associated with ischemia and can potentially be used to diagnose infarcted brain, myocardium, or ischemic muscles from peripheral vascular disease.

^{31}P NMR studies have been conducted to detect intracellular pH after renal transplant. A drop in intracellular renal pH as detected by ^{31}P NMR spectroscopy was found to be a bad prognostic sign. These techniques can be utilized to measure enzyme equilibrium and reaction kinetics as well.

^{13}C

The most recent nucleus to be studied by TMR is ^{13}C by utilizing an ^{1}H-decoupled ^{13}C spectrum. In nature 99% of carbon occurs as the isotope ^{12}C, which does not have a magnetic moment and therefore does not produce an NMR signal. The remaining 1% is the isotope ^{13}C, which does, however, give a spectrum rich in chemical information. Although ^{13}C NMR is relatively insensitive, compared to ^{1}H or ^{31}P, the wealth of chemical information that is available together with the possibility of increasing the natural abundance by administering ^{13}C-labeled metabolites compensate for the longer signal acquisition times that must be employed.

For example, molecules such as glucose can be labeled with ^{13}C, and subsequent NMR chemical analysis can detect the progress of the ^{13}C atom as it is distributed in the various carbon positions in the glucose molecule. The ^{13}C initially appears at the C1, C3, C4, and C5 position. The progress of the label enabled detailed metabolic pathways to be deduced.

Nuclear Magnetic Resonance Microscopy

With very high field strengths it may be possible to attain spatial resolution on the order of 10 micrometers. This opens the possibility of NMR chemical imaging at the microscopic level.

MEDICAL APPLICATION—A GREAT POTENTIAL

The capability of being able to image many nuclei, their two relaxation times, their state of flow, and the chemical shifts or metabolic events occurring around them offers an awesome potential for the diagnosis and treatment of human disease. The following discussion is by no means intended to indicate those potential applications that are currently present or even likely to be obtained within several decades, but merely a general framework within which to begin to consider the larger number of applications for this technology.

Conditions for which NMR Imaging Appears to be Superior to Existing Imaging Technology

Clinical studies, using NMR scanners in the 3 to 5 KG range and capable of 0.8 × 0.8 mm spatial resolution, have shown NMR imaging to be superior to CT scanning in imaging many pathological conditions in the brain and thorax.

NMR images are not prone to the aliasing and overrange artifacts that compromise the diagnostic utility of X-ray CT images and limit X-ray CT applications in the posterior fossa, temporal bone, and vertebral column (Fig. 1.3). The excellent contrast resolution eliminates the use of intravenous contrast media in most cases, and by using combinations of T_1-weighted inversion-recovery and T_2-weighted spin-echo techniques, edema can be separated from surrounding neoplastic tissue or blood (Fig. 6.4). NMR has been clearly shown to be superior to X-ray CT scanning in diagnosing demyelinating diseases, brain infarcts, congenital diseases, and some spinal column pathology (Figs. 8.2 to 8.7). NMR imaging has proved to be useful in evaluating normal biological events, such as the progressive myelinization of an infant's brain. A change in the normally expected level of myelinization for age indicates early brain pathology. Abnormalities of the bone marrow can best be evaluated by NMR imaging, as X-ray CT does not detect these tissues well. There are some cases in which benign neoplasms can be determined from malignant neoplasms, because benign neoplasms tend to have shorter T_1 images

---

FIG. 8.2. Transverse NMR scans of a patient with multiple sclerosis (*arrows*) using inversion-recovery (*left*) and spin-echo (*right*) techniques. Note the reversal in NMR signal from the multiple sclerosis lesions. Demyelinating processes in the brain such as multiple sclerosis are associated with an increase in water content and demyelinization. Since water protons are slow relaxing and lipid protons are fast relaxing, this increase in water content and decrease in lipid content causes a prolongation of both T_1 and T_2 relaxation times. Thus, the increasing water content and loss of myelin has a significant impact on the methodology employed in scanning these types of lesions as illustrated in this case in which the prolonged T_1 in T_1 weighted imaging sequences such as the inversion-recovery sequence in the left image results in a black or decreased NMR signal. Conversely, the prolonged T_2 causes an increase in NMR signal when the spin-echo or T_2 weighted imaging sequence is employed, which results in a very large NMR signal and white lesions as demonstrated on the right. This combination of effects makes NMR scanning superior to X-ray CT in detecting subtle changes in white matter demyelinating processes such as this case of multiple sclerosis. (Copyright Technicare Corporation. NMR image provided by courtesy of Technicare Corporation and the Cleveland Clinic Foundation.)

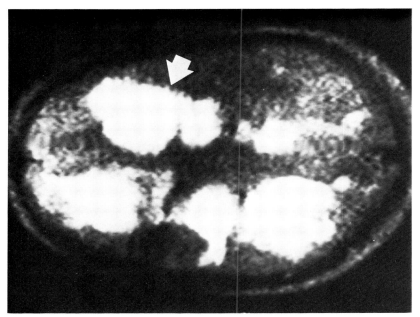

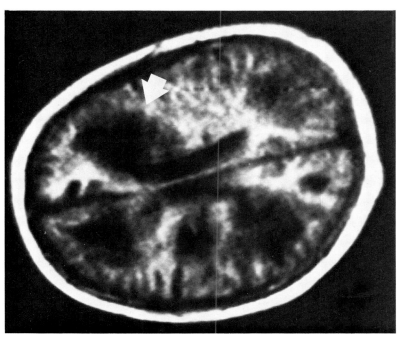

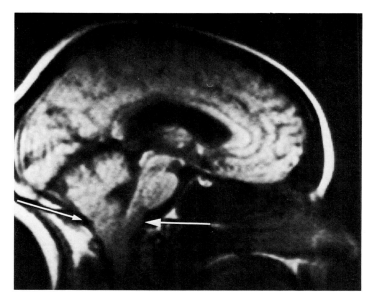

FIG. 8.3. Sagittal NMR scan of a patient with Arnold-Chiari malformation. Note the inferior projection of the cerebella tonsils (*arrows*). (Copyright Technicare Corporation. NMR image provided by courtesy of Technicare Corporation and the Cleveland Clinic Foundation.)

and those of malignant neoplasms tend to be somewhat longer (although there is considerable overlap in this area). But NMR is at least as good as CT in detecting lesions such as brain neoplasms and hydrocephalus.

In the mediastinum, fat has a very strong NMR signal, due to the comparatively shorter T_1 and longer T_2 with other mediastinal tissue; thus, other mediastinal masses are easily distinguishable from it. As opposed to CT, where hilar masses and large hilar blood vessels have similar electron density, due to the absence of NMR signal from rapidly flowing blood, large hilar blood vessels return no NMR signal and therefore, are easily distinguishable from the much stronger NMR signals from hilar neoplasms or granulomatous disease.

Applications of NMR in cardiovascular imaging are very promising (Fig. 8.8). By using different time intervals in inversion-recovery imaging sequences, the rate and direction of blood flow can be estimated, since slower flowing blood will cast a stronger NMR signal than the signal from more rapidly flowing blood, which is carried out of the scanning plane. Due to the atheromatous content of atherosclerotic plaques and the strong NMR signal returned from fat, ath-

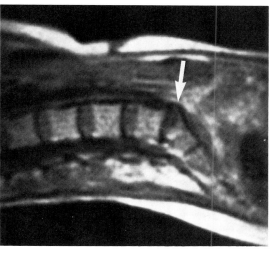

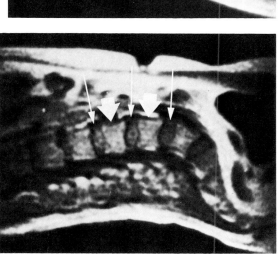

FIG. 8.4. Sagittal NMR scans of lumbar spine: (*left*): Normal: Disk (*long arrows*) and vertebral body (*short arrows*). The signal is from the bone marrow with the vertebral body; (*right*): Herniated L5, S1 disk (*arrow*). Note that the black structure anterior to the sacrum and lower lumbar vertebrae on these images is the bladder, which is seen as a black structure on the saturation-recovery images because of the prolonged T_1. This is due to the fact that very small molecules are suspended in the urine and that the energy transfer among the molecules is very inefficient thereby resulting in prolonged T_1 (and T_2) relaxation times. (Copyright Technicare Corporation. NMR image provided by courtesy of Technicare Corporation and the Cleveland Foundation.)

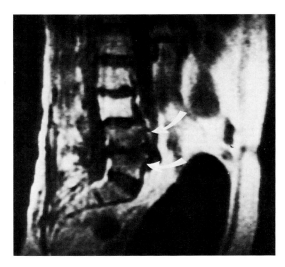

FIG. 8.4. continued. Degenerative disease with disruption of the bone marrow signal from L4 and L5 (*curved arrows*).

erosclerotic plaques stand out clearly against the rapidly flowing blood. In addition, as the vascular lumen is compromised, turbulence and/or slower flow begin to return a stronger NMR signal, indicating the degree of compromise of the vascular lumen. Care must be taken not to interpret turbulence as occlusion in this case as both would give a strong signal. Gated NMR scanning has shown great promise in detecting the edematous areas in and around infarcted myocardial tissue, and the early studies appear to be very promising for the general detection of vascular occlusion, and infarction or ischemia in the heart. Aortic dissections are well demonstrated on NMR images, due to the prominent flap present in the middle of the flowing blood on either side. In addition, the asymmetrical flow between the two channels is apparent. Systolic and diastolic blood flow can even be determined with the appropriate spin-echo technique, as an increased NMR signal (white) can be recorded from the aorta during diastole, whereas no signal is recorded during the systolic phase in which the blood is moving more rapidly.

NMR images of the abdomen are, in general, as good as those obtained from CT scanning, and certain liver metastases and fatty infiltration of the liver are more easily detected by NMR. However, at this point, NMR in abdominal diagnosis is not as clearly superior to other forms of imaging. Early studies have suggested that some

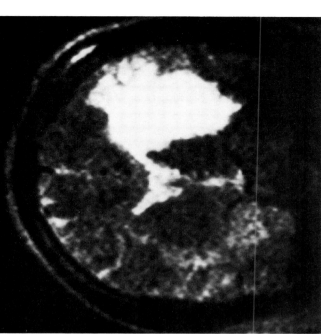

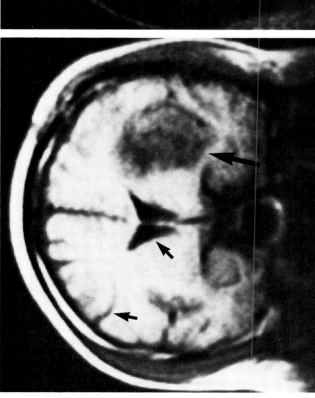

FIG. 8.5. Coronal NMR scans of a patient with a low-grade glioma (*long arrow*) using the saturation-recovery technique (*left*) and spin-echo technique (*right*). Note the shift from low to high NMR signal in both the neoplasm and cerebral spinal fluid in the ventricles and sulci (*short arrows*). Although a wide range of relaxation times exist, prolongation of T_1 and T_2 is associated with neoplastic disease and the T_1 saturation-recovery image thus demonstrates the prolonged T_1 of the neoplasm as a low signal or gray-black area, whereas the T_2 weighted spin-echo imaging sequence utilizes the prolongation of T_2 and demonstrates the associated increased NMR signal as a white lesion. Prolongation of both T_1 and T_2 in the cerebral spinal fluid is the reason for the similar change in the CSF in the sulci and cerebral ventricles. (Copyright Technicare Corporation. NMR image provided by courtesy of Technicare Corporation and the University Hospitals of Cleveland.)

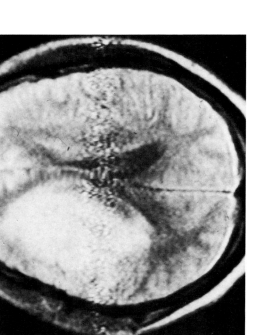

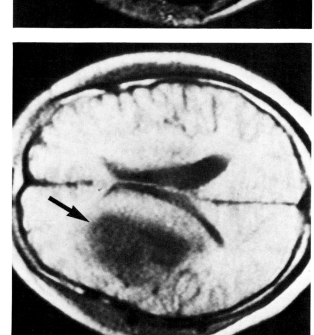

FIG. 8.6. A cross-sectional 0.3 T NMR scan of a patient with an astrocytoma (*arrow*): (*left*) Saturation recovery with a 0.5-sec delay; (*right*) Saturation recovery with a 2.0-sec delay. Note that the relatively short 0.5-sec interpulse delay in the top left figure is too short for the T₁ relaxation associated with the astrocytoma to have relaxed and therefore gives an attenuated or decreased NMR signal in the gray-black range. When further relaxation of T₁ is allowed using the 2.0-sec interpulse delay, the neoplasm is seen as a larger (white) NMR signal due to the increased proton density of the edema associated with the tumor. The black lesion in inversion recovery is again seen because of the prolonged T₁ in the tumor. Conversely, the large (white) signal from the lesion in the spin-echo T₂ weighted sequence is related to its prolonged T₂ relaxation time when compared to the surrounding tissues. (Copyright Technicare Corporation. NMR image provided by courtesy of Technicare Corporation and the Cleveland Clinic Foundation.)

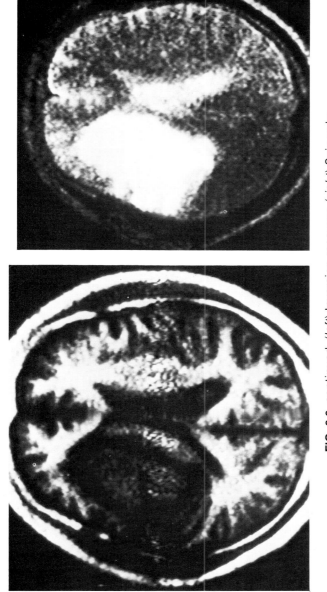

FIG. 8.6. continued. (*left*) Inversion-recovery; (*right*) Spin-echo.

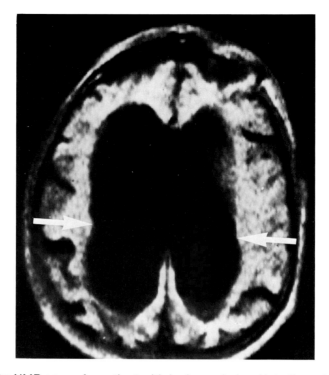

FIG. 8.7. An NMR scan of a patient with hydrocephalus. Note the enlarged sulci and ventricles (*arrows*). (Copyright Technicare Corporation. NMR image provided by courtesy of Technicare Corporation and the Cleveland Clinic Foundation.)

degree of tissue characterization and separation between normal, benign, and abnormal tissues can be obtained by determining T_1 and T_2 relaxation times. NMR joint and breast scanning is possible but efficacy has not been established. Because of the high information content of the NMR signal a color display may be preferable. And, since the NMR signal is *not* based on tissue density a gray scale may be misleading.

NMR spectroscopy has also been used in clinical diagnosis and spatial encoding of spectroscopy information will expand greatly the application of this variety of information. McArdle's syndrome has been diagnosed by detecting the extremely low intracellular pH at rest and after exercise in a patient in England. The fatty infiltration of the muscles in patients with muscular dystrophy is seen as an increase in the peak, due to $(CH_2)N$ in extremity scanning, and this has been used clinically to evaluate the progression of disease and effects of therapy. Naturally occurring ^{13}C spectra from human ex-

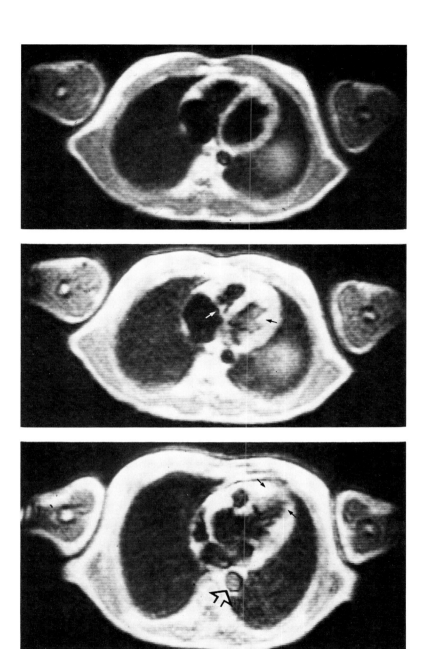

FIG. 8.8. Gated NMR cardiac scan of a normal patient in diastole (*top*) and systole (*middle*). Note the closure of the tricuspid valve (*white arrow*) and the appearance of the papillary muscle in the ventricular cavity (*black arrow*), and (*bottom*) a patient with a myocardial infarction and apical defect in the myocardium (*arrows*). Note the increase in NMR signal obtained from the aorta during diastole in the patient with myocardial infarction as compared to the other images due to the decreased cardiac output and slower flow in the patient with the infarction. (Copyright Technicare Corporation. NMR image provided by courtesy of Technicare Corporation and the Cleveland Clinic Foundation.)

tremities are known to come mainly from neutral triglycerides in fat tissues and provide information about nutritional fat deficiency and fatty infiltration in muscular dystrophy as well. A more important application medically, of course, is to enrich the ^{13}C environment with a labeled tracers and follow the labeled carbon through the metabolic cycles. Nunally has reported a widening of the phosphocreatine spectral line in association with adriamycin cardiac toxicity induced in rodents. Spatially encoding this type of information could eliminate the current diagnostic approach for assessing adriamycin toxicity (i.e., myocardial biopsy).

Conditions for which NMR Imaging Appears to be Inferior to Current Imaging Modalities

NMR imaging is not superior to current imaging techniques in all cases. The image is severely degraded by motion, and therefore, imaging lung nodules or intrinsic lesions in the gastrointestinal (GI) tract is difficult, due to the biological motion. The NMR signal from solids, i.e., cortical bone, is very weak (Fig. 8.9), and consequently, NMR is not useful in evaluating patients suspected of having renal or biliary calculi. Similarly, abnormalities of bone mineral, may not be visualized with NMR imaging, and certain neoplasms, which have calcifications associated with them, such as breast cancer and mucin-producing carcinomas of the bowel, may be more difficult to detect (Fig. 8.10). In addition, the NMR imaging systems are expensive and metallic life-support systems cannot be used around them, thus imaging patients from intensive-care units, or requiring other life-support systems may be difficult. Nevertheless, in general, this is a relatively safe, extremely powerful diagnostic modality, which is in all likelihood ultimately to be the diagnostic imaging modality of choice in most cases.

CONTRAST AGENTS

There are three basic parameters that can be changed to influence the images. These are: (a) the number of nuclei of interest, i.e., nuclear density; (b) the spin-lattice relaxation time characterizing the interaction of a nucleus with its environment (T_1); and (c) the spin-spin relaxation time, which describes the interaction of a nucleus and surrounding nuclei of the same kind (T_2). Images obtained using these parameters will differ from one another according to the tissue char-

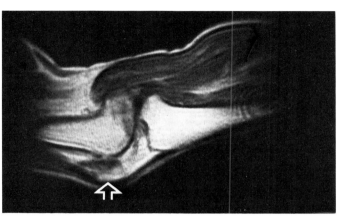

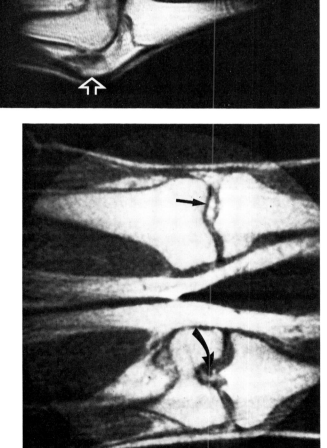

FIG. 8.9. An NMR scans through normal knee joints (*left*) and foot (*right*). Note the left lateral miniscus (*black straight arrow*), the cruciate ligaments (*curved black arrow*), the patella (*open arrows*). (Copyright Technicare Corporation. NMR image (*left*) provided by courtesy of Technicare Corporation. Copyright Fonar Corporation. NMR fmage (*right*) provided courtesy of Fonar Corporation.)

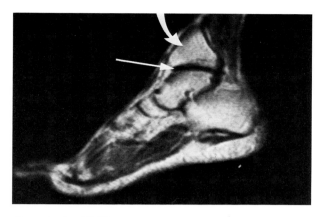

FIG. 8.9. continued. An NMR scan through the foot. Note the black cortical bone (*straight arrow*) and marrow (*curved arrow*) of the tarsal bones. NMR Image provided courtesy of Fonar Corporation.

acteristics. The best nuclei for NMR imaging in human tissues are determined by the intrinsic sensitivity of the nuclei and the concentration in mammalian tissue. Thus, in human tissues, NMR imaging utilizing ^1H, ^{14}N, ^{31}P, will produce images of higher quality than those produced using other resonating atoms.

The development of NMR contrast agents can be approached from one of these three aspects. First, a change in the natural abundance or concentration (selectively) of a given atom in an abnormal or normal tissue can be produced. In this regard, the higher the intrinsic sensitivity of the nucleus and the more selectively concentrated, the better the NMR contrast agent will be. Secondly, by using paramagnetic atoms, one can attempt to influence the relaxation times of nuclei normally used in NMR imaging (i.e., ^1H, T_1, and T_2 signals). Finally, one can utilize NMR projection imaging, which will decrease the duration of NMR imaging to the millisecond level, and thus will allow the imaging of moving structures and also the imaging of atoms with very long relaxation times. Electron paramagnetic resonance (EPR) and the use of topical magnetic resonance spectroscopy with surface coils may also exploit these types of contrast agents.

Increasing Natural Abundance

Fluorine has a very high NMR signal sensitivity. In general, fluorine is not useful in NMR imaging because its natural abundance is

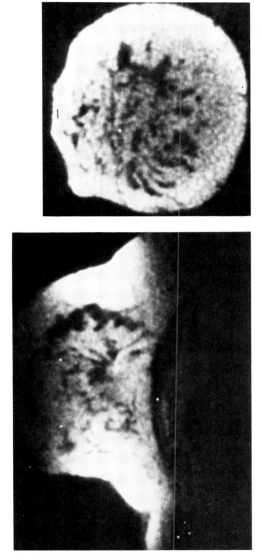

FIG. 8.10. Sagittal (*left*) and cross-sectional (*right*) NMR scan of a normal breast. (Copyright Technicare Corporation. NMR image provided by courtesy of Technicare Corporation.)

relatively low. Fluorine compounds have been used, however, as artificial blood substitutes for their oxygen-carrying potential, and perhaps more importantly for NMR imaging, fluorine emulsions have been shown to concentrate around neoplastic and abscess lesions. Thus, the fluorine molecule, in sufficient concentrations, could be directly imaged, and since the biological prevalence is so low, large accumulations of fluorine nuclei would indicate the presence of either abnormal neoplastic or abscess tissue. Another element, copper (^{63}Cu), is also an attractive NMR contrast agent because of its ability to be targeted to the liver and because it is chelated by macromolecules like transferrin, which has been shown to collect in some neoplasms.

Altering Relaxation Time

One class of paramagnetic agents that appear promising as NMR contrast agents are the piperidine derivatives. A nitroxide stable free radical has been successfully tested by Brash in animals. Nitroxide stable free radicals are paramagnetic and demonstrate relatively strong proton relaxation enhancement, due to an unpaired electron in one of the orbits. The unpaired electron promotes both spin-spin and spin-lattice relaxation of the surrounding protons—in other words, T_1 and T_2 decrease. This results in an increase in the intensity in the T_1 weighted NMR signal from tissues labeled with the free radical. The proton relaxation enhancement of the nitroxide stable free radical is comparable to that from cupric (Cu^{2+}) and ferrous (Fe^{2+}) ions in similar concentrations. Using ESR spectroscopy, the concentration of this agent *in vivo* in biological tissues can be assessed. This contrast agent has successfully shown experimentally induced unilateral hydronephrosis, renal ischemia, and renal vein thrombosis, which were not apparent prior to contrast enhancement. In addition, the NMR contrast resolution brain inflammation has been increased after stable free radical administration.

pH Alteration

Using NMR spectroscopy, investigators at Oxford University have found that the inorganic ^{31}P changes according to the pH of the surroundings. The pH of malignant tissue is generally lower than that of normal tissue and, in addition, can be lowered significantly by the systemic administration of bicarbonate or the regional administration of dilute acids. Thus, topical magnetic resonance with or without local acidification of the malignant neoplasm could potentially be a technique of achieving "contrast enhancement" by altering the resonant frequency of naturally present, cancer-based inorganic phosphorous.

O_2 and Hypoxic Cells

Molecular oxygen is also paramagnetic. Malignant tissue is distinctive in that it contains hypoxic cells. It is likely that increasing the PO_2 of blood in general will significantly enhance ^1H relaxation and change the proton signal (as described below). This may be very useful in detecting not only malignant tissue but perhaps abscesses as well.

Blood Flow

Because blood is moving, conventional cross-sectional NMR imaging does not receive an NMR signal from the blood vascular space. Thus, blood vessels appear as an absence or lack of NMR signal. Utilizing projection NMR imaging with the capability of obtaining data in milliseconds, one could perhaps perform NMR "angiography" without contrast media. However, fluorine, in the form of perfluorinated hydrocarbon emulsions has been demonstrated to be relatively biologically safe. Injection of a small amount of fluorine, which remains within the vascular space, would markedly increase the native fluorine signal, which could be subsequently imaged in a projection mode. In this regard, it could be useful in imaging intrinsic vascular lesions.

In addition, the Hammersmith Group in England has shown that the signal strength from intraventricular blood will be enhanced as the O_2 content of blood is increased, and that tissues perfused with higher concentrations of O_2 will produce stronger signals than when perfused with lower O_2 concentrations. Therefore, it appears that paramagnetics, such as oxygen, may be used to enhance the difference between diseased and nondiseased tissue. Another paramagnetic element, manganese (Mn), has also been shown to be useful in detecting areas of decreased perfusion, since it distributes in proportion to blood flow. The ability to monitor the intravascular space with a blood pool agent like perfluorinated compounds or to monitor the physiological accumulation of paramagnetic agents like oxygen or manganese, has extensive implications for the diagnosis of congenital or acquired cardiovascular disease.

The phenomenon of relaxation has an effect on blood flow imaging. Assume blood flows through a vessel perpendicular to the imaging plane at a velocity v and further that the pulse sequence used is inversion-recovery with both inversion and detection pulse being slice-selective. During the recovery period of t seconds, the "magnetically tagged" blood in the cylindrical element of length x cm (slice thickness) has advanced by length $L = v.t$. Under certain timing and flow conditions it is evident that some of the detected signal arises from in flowing blood protons which are unaffected by the inversion pulse and thus provide a larger NMR signal following the 90° RF_x pulse, resulting in enhanced brightness when compared to a stationary situation. Using similar arguments, the spin echo sequence invokes a diminution of the pixel value if flow is present because the in-coming precessing protons are out of phase. It is to be anticipated that refinement of these methods will soon permit the clinician to obtain an accurate estimate of blood flow.

Chapter 9

Nuclear Magnetic Resonance Imaging Systems

The learning curve for NMR has been greatly shortened by the previous experience with CT scanners. Whereas the tremendous diagnostic potential of CT was relatively slowly appreciated, the tendency for imaging specialists to speculate generously about the potential applications of NMR are testified not only by the large number of attendees at NMR scientific sessions but also the large number of equipment manufacturers that have entered into the field very early. It is not only the scientific applications that are driving this enthusiasm, however. Many who were kept out of the CT field by federal regulations are determined not be left out this time. In addition, because of the absence of ionizing radiation, there is no *a priori* recognition by other nonradiologist physicians of a control restriction on this technology. Also, the progress of NMR imaging has been a rapid one. Although clinical images had been shown as early as 1976, a major improvement in the quality and detail of NMR human images has ocurred since 1980, following the introduction of superconducting magnet technology into these systems. The superconducting magnets are superior because of higher magnetic field strength, thereby improving signal-to-noise ratio (creating a less noisy picture and allowing shorter imaging times) and better field uniformity (allowing better reproduction of anatomic detail in the image) compared to previous resistive NMR units. However, images from resistive NMR scanners have also greatly improved.

Recently, two new developments have rejuvenated the enthusiasm for NMR. Proton images obtained at relatively high imaging field strengths of above 1T have been demonstrated, which suggests that both proton imaging and perhaps imaging spectroscopy can be done with the same imaging system without having to either have two magnets for these two projects or change field strength from one demand to the other (Fig 9.1). In addition, several companies are in the process of making or developing permanent magnet systems precluding the need for large power supplies and/or cryogenics. Political, scientific, and economic arguments can be made in favor of different aspects of these systems, and only time will determine the eventual evolution of this technology.

TYPES OF SCANNERS

Permanent, Resistive, and Superconducting Magnets

The components for an NMR imaging system are fairly well defined, although there will undoubtedly be modifications of each of these units as time progresses. A large magnet is used to impose a strong, external, and relatively uniform magnetic field. Within the aperture of the magnet are a series of current-carrying gradient coils that modify the uniform, external field, and these gradient coils are used to spatially encode the NMR signal. Next, a transmitter is connected to a radio-frequency transmitter-received antenna with which the RF pulse is broadcast into and received from the sample or object being scanned. The signal is then amplified, filtered, digitized, and processed by a computer for image construction and display functions (see Apendix II).

There are two general types of magnets: permanent magnets and magnets that are produced by electric current, which produces the

---

FIG. 9.1. An NMR proton scan obtained at a field strength of 1.5 T (*top, left and right*) and a phosphorus spectrum (*bottom*) obtained from the same scanner. The significance of this image is that a proton image can be obtained at this field strength under any conditions. It was previously felt that attentuation of high-frequency RF signals would preclude imaging at these levels. The fact that it can be performed suggests that with one scanner operating at a high field strength, hydrogen and perhaps phosphorus imaging can be performed. This may also indicate the possibility of doing chemical shift hydrogen imaging as well.

These axial images (*top*) were acquired on a 1.5-T NMR system, operating at 1.5 T using a partial saturation technique with a 400-msec interpulse delay. The slices are 20 mm. These were the first NMR images at 1.5 T (63 MH$_z$). The P-31 spectra was also obtained on the 1.5-T superconducting magnet whole body size bore system. This is the first ever *in vivo* spectra of a human head (normal volunteer). (Copyright The General Electric Company images, supplied courtesy of the Medical College of Wisconsin.)

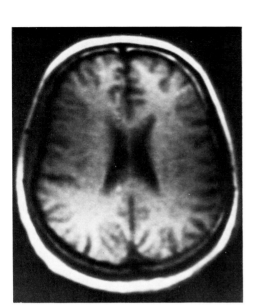
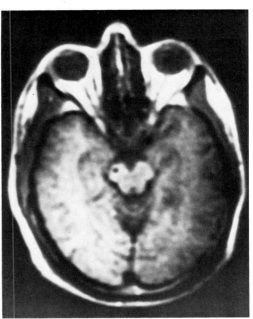
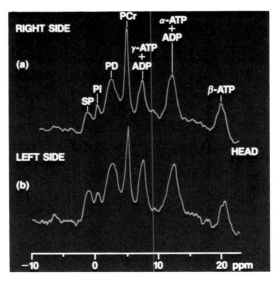

magnetic field around the conductor. There are, in general, two types of magnets that use electric current depending on the type of core—iron core and air core. An iron-core magnet consists of a large central metal C- or H-shaped block of iron with multiple turns of a resistive conductor (usually copper or aluminum) wrapped around it. These wires may also be suspended in air creating a so-called air-core magnet. There are essentially two kinds of air-core magnets—resistive air-core magnets and superconducting air-core magnets. Resistive air-core magnets are operated at room temperature and require a constant power source to maintain the magnetic field in the current-carrying conductors. In the superconducting air-core magnet, the current-carrying conductors are made of niobium-titanium (NbTi) embedded in a copper matrix. The conductor is submerged in liquid helium that in turn is surrounded by a vacuum, a subsequent layer of liquid nitrogen, then another vacuum, and finally insulation. The copper matrix for the NbTi conductors protect the system from destruction in case of accidental quench (i.e., a loss of superconductivity). When running at superconducting temperatures ($4°$ K), the copper serves as a heat conductor but not as an electrical conductor, while the NbTi, which has no resistance, conducts the current. If the temperature begins to rise, however, the copper quickly becomes the less resistive of the two conductors and safely dissipates the current previously confined to the NbTi conductors, preventing melting of these wire filaments.

Permanent magnets have some major drawbacks in that they are sensitive to changes in temperature, very heavy and surface scratches on bits of metal destroy field homogeneity; nevertheless, permanent magnet systems eliminate many of the problems that arise with superconducting or resistive magnets. With permanent magnets there is no potential for quenching nor any special power requirements. There is minimal fringe field and limited missile effect, so site selection is a much less significant problem. There are no costly cyrogenic expenses, and there are no moving parts except for the motorized patient cot. Currently, the price of these systems is comparable to superconducting magnets. The one major concern is field homogeneity and low field strength in these systems, and they have yet to be widely tested. Their maintenance would be substantially less than that of any other system. Thus, the advantages of permanent magnets rests in the area of very low maintenance and little cost in site preparation.

A resistive magnet creates a magnetic field by passing an electric current through a wire wrapped around a core. The larger the current and the greater the number of turns of wire, the greater the magnetic field created. The limit on magnetic field strength appears to be related primarily to the amount of heat that is dissipated by the current as it flows against the resistance of the wire. For useful fields, very large currents are required, e.g., 100 to 150 amp. In addition, the magnet creates such sufficient heat that it must be water cooled, which can require several liters of water/min. 1.5 KG magnetic fields can be obtained with resistive magnets, but at this point the power consumption, cooling requirements, and bulk (weight) of the magnet appear to make it unlikely to achieve higher fields with resistance systems. Above 1.5 KG the advantages are weighted in favor of the superconducting magnets. All the available evidence to date indicates that images created with fields in excess of 1.5 KG will be substantially superior to those obtained below 1.5 KG; therefore, the balance favors the superconducting NMR system. At the higher fields, the NMR signal strength and signal/noise increases, and the imaging time can be decreased. Once up to field strength, the superconducting magnet operates without using any additional electrical current. The large power consumption of resistive magnets is eliminated. The magnetic field can be maintained at a constant strength and with high uniformity—both important for improving image detail.

The magnets represent a substantial portion of the manufacturers cost of producing the superconducting system. For example, the cost of a 1.5 T magnet is about $750,000. Liquid helium and liquid nitrogen are required to maintain the low temperature of the magnet, ensuring superconductivity. These cryogens (especially helium) are not universally available and require special knowledge in handling. Furthermore, the cost of the cryogens (which require periodic replenishment) is a significant portion of the operating cost of a system.

Quenching, or the loss of the ability to maintain a high field in a superconducting state, can occur with collapse of the magnetic field. Quenching can also occur with a slow decay in the field, a slow increase in magnet temperature, and a boil-off of cryogens. Subsequently, cryogens will have to be replaced and magnetic field brought back up through recharging. A rapid decay in the field can also happen with rapid boil-off of liquid helium and possible permanent damage to the magnet. In addition, there may be a health hazard to personnel in the area from the liquid helium and nitrogen boil-off and possibly from the rapidly changing field. The cost of replenishing the cryogens is estimated to be as much as $15,000, similar to the replacement cost of an X-ray tube for a CT scanner. In a superconducting system, the magnetic field is always up to strength. The potential problem may be that someone inadvertently brings a ferrous or metallic object too close to the magnet and the object can be sucked into the magnet, where it will strike or stick to the side of the magnet with considerable force.

Resistive and superconducting magnet NMR imaging systems have been operational for several years, and permanent imaging systems are now available. The English were early leaders in NMR imaging technology but have lagged behind the more recent developments from the United States. The best images to date have been obtained with the highest field strength systems. These images provide image quality comparable to existing X-ray CT scanners with a wealth of information—sometimes the information is superior to X-ray CT, at other times it is complementary or inferior. NMR images are both diagnostic and in some situations provide better information than other modalities, specifically X-ray CT. In addition, there is no doubt that there will be cases in which X-ray CT is superior to NMR (e.g., bone imaging). At present, most interest is focused on how NMR compares to X-ray CT in areas where CT is well established (e.g., brain imaging). However, it is most likely that there will be a large class of examinations for which NMR is uniquely suited and for which X-ray CT is not appropriate. For example, NMR seems to be useful for imaging soft tissues like tendons and ligaments that are usually not identified with X-ray CT. Another prime area will be visualizing blood vessels without contrast media and evaluation of blood flow disorders. Tissue characterization is an exciting application of NMR, due to the richness of the NMR signal.

Future Trends

NMR imaging is still evolving rapidly. It is not clear what magnetic field strength is optimal for imaging. Originally, it was felt that 1.5 KG was maximum for body imaging. Now that 3.5 KG images are not only feasible, but superior, many believe that 5 KG will be even better. Over 1.0 T images offer the exciting possibility of chemical shift imaging. At some point image quality diminishes based on the fact that radio-frequency signals required for NMR imaging are more highly attenuated and eddy currents from the gradient coils increase as field strength increases. From an installation viewpoint, it is important to recognize that system cost increases and site requirements become more complex at higher field strengths.

The trend toward higher field strength magnets (e.g., over 1.0 T) favors whole body NMR spectroscopy to detect alterations in metabolism based on changes in ^{1}H, ^{31}P, and/or ^{13}C NMR spectra and to increase patient through-put. Attempts to combine imaging with spectroscopy will represent important research efforts to maximize the information that NMR provides.

NMR fluoroscopy and projection imaging is on the horizon. Projection iron-core resistive NMR scanners with ±0.2 mm spatial resolution would be ideal for noninvasive imaging of coronary arteries, bypass grafts, and other blood vessels.

Equipment Currently Available

One of the indications of how much enthusiasm is being generated for NMR imaging technology is the large number of companies who have started manufacturing NMR systems. In addition to the ten companies listed below, Toshiba Medical Systems, Medi Q, Inc., Synergetics, Inc., Universal Medical Scanners, Inc., Bruker, IBM and Starburst General, Inc. are advertising and/or demonstrating NMR images and scanners.

The commercial market for NMR imaging systems is quickly evolving. The number of companies currently designing and/or marketing NMR imaging systems appears to be as great as it was in the early days of CT. The following list of companies is only representative, and the information is meant only as a guide.

1. *Diasonics.* Diasonics acquired the rights to the NMR research that UCSF had developed (previously supported by Pfizer, Inc.). Diasonics is building up an NMR division to transfer the UCSF prototype technology (using a 3 KG magnet) into a series of additional systems for clinical trials. One advantage with the newer system is that the magnet will have a larger bore for patient access. It is unknown whether or not performance will be different with these new magnets.

2. *Elscint.* Elscint, an Israeli medical imaging company, displayed prototype images at the 1982 RSNA.

3. *Fonar.* Fonar was an early entrant in the NMR imaging business with a resistive NMR system. Their method for producing cross-

sectional images (Fonar) differs from later methods used by the other companies.

4. *General Electric (GE)*. GE has delivered to the University of Pennsylvania one resistive magnet imaging system (currently being installed); another resistive system is under collaborative development with Yale. They have a 15 KG superconducting magnet operational at their R/D center in Schenectady and are installing a 3 KG and, shortly thereafter, a 5 KG superconducting system at the factory in Milwaukee. The 3 KG system will be moved to the Medical College of Wisconsin sometime in 1983 and there will be several 5 KG systems in the 1983/1984 time frame. A 15 KG magnet will go to Duke University and Pennsylvania in 1983 under a collaborative agreement with GE. GE's management has made a major commitment to NMR, and announced a commercial product in 1983.

5. *Intermagnetics General (IGC)*. IGC is a producer of superconducting magnets. They are approaching the NMR imaging business by providing superconducting magnets and support technology. In addition, they are working on a very high field NMR imaging spectroscopy system for delivery in 1983.

6. *International Business Machines (IBM)*. IBM not only owns approximately 25% of Bruker, a leading concern in NMR spectroscopy, but is also interested in the NMR imaging market. They are sponsoring work at Harvard and the Massachusetts Institute of Technology (National Magnet Laboratory) and have an in-house NMR research and development program.

7. *Picker (GEC)*. GEC of Great Britain has acquired Picker. GEC initially had the technology of one of the English NMR groups, at the University of Nottingham (a resistive system), and acquired the Hammersmith superconducting NMR technology from EMI. The insuperconducting system is expected to operate at 2.5 to 3.0 KG.

8. *Philips*. Philips showed their early resistive magnet images in 1981. They have ordered a 15 KG magnet from Intermagnetics General, a competitor of Oxford Instruments for superconducting magnets. Philips will investigate phosphorous imaging spectroscopy with this NMR scanner.

9. *Siemens*. Siemens has had a longstanding NMR research program in Erlangen and has created images using a resistive system. They now have a 5 KG magnet for an initial superconducting prototype system.

10. *Technicare*. Technicare is a subsidiary of Johnson and Johnson. Technicare has had a 1.5 KG resistive unit in operation at the Massachusetts General Hospital. They also have a 3.5 KG superconducting system. Technicare's original focus was on the resistive technology, because of its lower price and easier site preparations. However, Technicare offers an upgrade option to a superconducting magnet anytime within the first two years of operation, and they offer magnets over 1.5 T field strength.

Chapter 10

Hazards and Site Planning

Medical diagnosis utilizing NMR scanners may be one of the first diagnostic modalities in which there is more risk for the operators of the equipment than for the patients (Fig. 10.1). To date, no adverse effects attributable to imaging have been observed in patients or volunteers. The major risk to NMR system operators comes from the large magnetic fields associated with these devices. Any metallic object can become a potentially lethal projectile in close proximity to the strong magnetic fields. To avoid this problem, all imaging units are guarded by metallic detectors similar to those used for screening airports and other public places. However, the sensitivity in NMR scanning units is set extremely low and many false alarms occur; they often discharge spontaneously, and after some time personnel tend to ignore the signals. This lack of vigilance can potentially produce significant consequences. An unexpected risk of Gaussian carditis was reported in the August 12, 1982 issue of the *New England Journal of Medicine*. Credit cards are not metallic and therefore do not affect metallic sensors; however, credit cards can be demagnetized and consequently will not work in any system requiring a metallic code to be present. To avoid this embarrassment, the removal of not only all metallic objects but all credit cards as well is advised.

One major advantage of NMR imaging systems, when compared with CT scanners, is that patients are not exposed to ionizing radiation. There is no evidence at the moment to suggest that there is a health hazard from the presently utilized imaging techniques. Nevertheless, patients are exposed to relatively intense static, gradient, and radio-frequency induced magnetic fields, and the possibility that either early or late adverse effects from exposure must be considered.

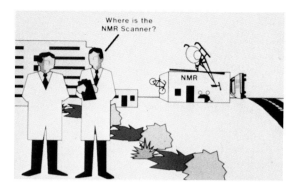

FIG. 10.1. (NMR cartoon).

MAGNETIC FIELDS

Most of the data accumulated regarding static magnetic fields has been accumulated in animals at the 1 T level. A small electrical potential in the large blood vessels that is generated by the flow of blood perpendicular to the magnetic field has been observed. Theoretically, if the flow potential were sufficiently large, it could affect the heart either by direct stimulation or by indirect stimulation of the pressure receptors situated in the aortic arch or carotid bodies. But even at static fields up to 10 T, no adverse effects on squirrel monkey ECGs have been recorded. Mutogenic effects in mammals have been studied in both static magnetic fields (T_1) and gradient fields with no adverse effect demonstrated on either adult or embryonic rodents. Extensive data have been accumulated by the National Institute for Occupational Safety and Health and the World Health Organization as well as the State Department in conjunction with employees who were exposed to high levels of microwave radiation at the Moscow Embassy, and no evidence of leukemia or other carcinogenesis has been recorded. Nevertheless, Milham reported in the July 22, 1982 issue of the *New England Journal of Medicine* an increased incidence of mortality due to leukemia in men occupationally exposed to electrical and magnetic fields in Washington State from 1950 to 1979. These observations have yet to be confirmed by other studies. No adverse effects from magnetic fields have been reported from personnel working in linear accelerators or high-energy physics labs. These individuals experience exposures of up to 2 T for short periods of time.

Gradient magnetic fields are pulsed and therefore have a time-varying component that will induce electrical currents in body tissues. Sufficiently intense flux densities could potentially stimulate electrically excitable cells, which would include nerve cells and muscle fibers of the heart and respiratory musculature. The most sensitive response of the body is the stimulation of the retina resulting in the sensation of flashes of light from stimulation of the magnetic retinal phosphenes. In man, this threshold has a minimum value of 2 to 3 $Tsec^{-1}$ at 20 to 50 Hz. Most other tissues in the body appear to be much less sensitive. Rodents have been exposed to pulse fields where the maximum rate of change was 60 $Tsec^{-1}$ with pulse rates as rapid as 60 msec with no effect having been seen on heart rate, blood pressure, or respiratory rate even after one hour of exposure (J. Gore & Associates, personal communication). The typical values used in routine clinical imaging range from between 0.04 $Tsec^{-1}$ and 5 $Tsec^{-1}$, although a few subjects have experienced rates of changes high as 20 $Tsec^{-1}$.

RADIO-FREQUENCY MAGNETIC FIELD

Electrical currents induced in the body by exposure to radio-frequency fields are not able to excite nervous tissue. The effects of high-energy RF are confined to heating, due to resistive losses of energy in the tissues. This is a principle used in short-wave diathermy therapy. In general, chronic exposure to radio-frequency power densities producing an average power deposition of approximately 1 Wkg^{-1} is considered safe, from a heat production point of view with a peak deposition of 8 Wkg^{-1} in any gram of tissue. This power deposition is roughly equivalent to a person's basic metabolic rate, and if no heat were lost from the body, it would raise tissue temperature about 1°C in an hour. Tissues with poor blood supply, and therefore decreased rates of cooling, experience greater elevations of temperature. Those tissues with no blood supply, like the lens of the eye, or poor blood supply, like the testes, could be regarded as target organs for heat sensitivity. Generally, the maximum time average absorbed power deposition during NMR imaging is substantially less than 1 Wkg^{-1}. Therefore, this does not appear to be a problem. Metallic surgical clips or large prostheses could absorb more heat than body tissues.

The effect on artificial pacemakers of the magnetic field used in

NMR is not known. Many manufacturers of pacemakers include reed relays within the pacemaker to provide a means of altering the pacemaker operation with an external magnet, which is placed on the outside of the body. Magnetic field strengths ranging from 10 to 50 G will activate the relays in a pacemaker, and thus, any patients with these types of pacemakers should not be allowed to encounter field strengths of over 3 to 5 G. In practical terms, this means that no patients should be allowed in corridors one or two floors above or below the NMR scanner at a comparable distance on either side. Interference by very weak magnetic fields can cause some modern trigger pacemakers to reverse to an asynchronous mode, and because of these concerns people with pacemakers or large metal implants have not been scanned in NMR systems.

In conclusion, the evidence from animal experiments involving exposure to high magnetic fields and the limited studies of human patients and volunteers exposed to clinical NMR imaging systems suggest that the fields used in the present systems are well below threshold for any adverse biological effect. Unless the requirement for magnetic field strength and RF power input greatly exceed the current expectations, the risk to patients undergoing magnetic resonance scanning is likely to be substantially less than for that encountered with radiographic equipment. Hazards and risks are more likely to be greater for those individuals working with the equipment or passing near it. The potential hazards resulting from the use of magnetic resonance imaging equipment are thus related to the following general areas: (a) injuries from ferromagnetic objects accelerated by large static magnetic fields; (b) effects on pacemakers, protheses, and any equipment using cathode-ray tubes (CRT) that are near the magnetic field; (c) biological effects of static magnetic field, induced currents from rapid changes in magnetic field, and heating from RF fields.

SITE PLANNING HAZARDS

A major consideration in the decision to have an NMR imaging facility is the architectural requirements. The structural, mechanical, electrical, and spatial requirements of the system must be carefully evaluated with respect to whether the stem will be placed in an existing building or a building that was specially built for NMR imaging. Difficulty in making these determinations is that there are still several significant unknowns in NMR technology. Investigators are still evaluating the optimal field strength for imaging applications. Without the answer to this question and others essential to optimal system design, it is impossible to predict the ideal configuration of the clinical systems that will be developed in the future. Nevertheless, certain fundamental characteristics of NMR imaging suites, specifically very strong magnetic fields and a radio-frequency transmitter-receiver, impose definite constraints on the architecture of an NMR suite. This section is designed to serve as a guideline only, and each group will require special assistance to fit the NMR imager selected into the space available. Nevertheless, a general outline of the problems and questions to be encountered should be useful.

Aside from engineering concerns, the general questions to be evaluated in NMR site planning are:

1. What will be the effect of the magnetic field on personnel and equipment in the immediate environment?
2. What will be the effect of metallic structures, vehicles, and electrical equipment on the NMR system itself?

The static magnetic field of any NMR system is three-dimensional and extends above and below the magnet as well as into the surrounding space on the same level. In addition, the field is not circular and extends further in the direction of the magnet board than perpendicular to the long axis. The magnetic field, nevertheless, falls off as the cube of the distance from the magnet system. For those planning a two-magnet suite with an imaging magnet in combination with a spectroscopy system, the best overall approach is to align the magnets perpendicular to each other to decrease the total overall field area.

The large three-dimensional magnetic field created by the NMR magnet is the major limiting factor in system location, especially if it is to go into an existing building. There are magnetic materials in the immediate environment that can distort the magnetic field of the system, degrading image quality and making NMR spectroscopy and/or ESR spectroscopy impossible. As mentioned, the magnetic field can interfere with the function of certain mechanical and/or electrical devices such as cathode-ray tubes and patients' pacemakers, and these magnetic field effects must be carefully considered and minimized if possible.

In this regard, the intended ultimate purpose of the imaging system is critically important. If a basic clinical unit capable of proton density imaging is all that is required, then a 0.15 T resistive system will suffice and site selection will be much simpler. However, if chemical shift spectroscopy and perhaps hydrogen density imaging as well is required, then at least a 1.5 T magnet strength will be required and greatly complicate the architectural design and controlled space.

For purposes of illustration of the kinds of concerns and problems to be faced in site preparation, a site model and field strength lines are presented for a 0.5 T superconducting magnet—field strengths and imaging suite design for the same plane as the magnet (Fig 10.2) and field strengths encountered in the plane perpendicular to the magnet's long axis (Fig. 10.3). Table 10.1 lists some of the influences of the external environment on the magnetic field. Table 10.2 lists some influences of the magnetic field on the external environment, and Table 10.3 some structural aspects of a hypothetical suite. Once again, however, these are meant only to indicate the general approach to site preparation; the actual design will vary from manufacturer to manufacturer.

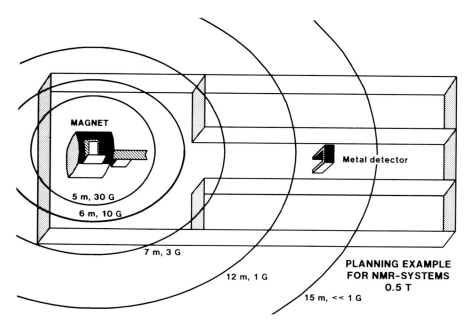

FIG. 10.2. Fringe field, planning example for a 0.5 T superconducting NMR magnet. Fringe field in the long axis.

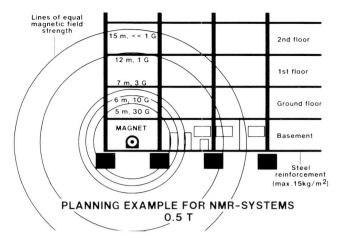

FIG. 10.3. Fringe field in the transverse axis.

TABLE 10.1. *External influences on the magnetic field minimum distance[a]*

1 m Distance
Steel reinforcement in ceiling and floor; 15 kg Fe/m^2

5 m Distance
Steel girders, highly reinforced concrete columns and beams

12 m Distance
Hospital transportation systems (bed transport, conveyance equipment)

12 m Distance
Very strong HF-generators

15 m Distance
Elevators, vehicles (trucks, cars)

15 m Distance
Power cables, transformers

[a] Distance equals to the center of the magnet.

TABLE 10.2. *Influence of the magnetic field on nearby equipment minimum distance[a]*

5 m Distance
Computers

7 m Distance
Television equipment, monitor screen

6 m Distance
Pacemaker perpendicular to the axis of the magnet

8.3 m Distance
Pacemaker along the axis of the magnet

15 m Distance
X-ray unit with image intensifier nuclear-medicine (gamma camera)

[a] Distance equals from the center of the magnet.

TABLE 10.3. *Structural aspects*

Weights and Dimensions (0.5 T S/C magnet)		Transport Path		Maximum Component Weight	
NMR magnet, filled	5300 kg	Minimum floor width	2.50 m	NMR magnet	4800 kg
Dimensions (l × w × h)	2,3 m × 2 m × 2.54 m	Minimum floor height	2.80 m	He can	460 kg
Patient couch	300 kg	Minimum door width	2.50 m	N can	800 kg
Dimensions (l × w × h)	3.0 m × 0.67 m × 0.65 m	Minimum door height	2.80 m		
Recommended size of room for magnet	10 m × 10 m				
Minimum size of room for magnet	5 m × 8 m				
Minimum room height	3.5 m				

TABLE 10.4. *Typical magnet specifications*

Type	0.13 T permanent magnet	0.15 T resistive	0.3 T S/C	0.5 T S/C	1.5–2.0 T S/C	Gradient coil power supply
Size (length × height)	25' × 10' (standard shielded room size)	6.9' × 7.5' (2.1 m × 2.3 m)	7.5' × 8.2' (2.3 m × 2.5 m)	7.5' × 8.2' (2.3 m × 2.5 m)	7.5' × 9.8' (2.3 m × 3.0 m)	2.6' × 5.9' (0.8 m × 1.8 m)
Weight	1,000 tons	9020 lb max (4100 kg) 5500 lb typical (2500 kg)	8800 lb (400 kg) 9900 lb[b] (4500 kg)	9460 lb (4300 kg) 10,560 lb (4800 kg)	16,500 lb (7550 kg) 17,710 lb[b] (8050 kg)	1100 lb (500 kg)
Minimum ceiling height	10'	9.5' (2.9 m)	9.5' (2.9 m)	9.5' (2.9 m)	14' (4.2 m)	N/A
Magnetic field distance[a] (3 gauss/1 gauss)	None (outside shielded room)	21' (6.4 m)/ 31' (9.4 m)	27' (8.2 m)/ 37' (11.9 m)	33' (10 m)/ 47' (14.3 m)	45' (13.7 m)/ 67' (20.4 m)[d]	N/A
Maximum power demand	None[c]	85 KVA max 60 KVA typical 3 phase	25 KVA max 3 phase	25 KVA max 3 phase	25 KVA max 3 phase	15 KVA to 75 KVA
Cooling requirements	Room air conditioning	Water: 95 liters/min (Magnet + power supply)	LN_2: 2 liters/hr LHe: 0.5 liters/hr H_2O: 3 liters/min[e]	LN_2: 2 liters/hr LHe: 0.5 liters/hr H_2O: 5 liters/min[a]	LN_2: 2 liters/hr LHe: 0.5 liters/hr H_2O: 10 liters/min[e]	H_2O: 10 liters/min coil 10 liters/min (power supply)

Sources: General Electric and Fonar.

[a] s/c = superconducting magnets; [b] with cryogens; [c] electrical supply to room 40 kw; [d] for 1.5 T field strength; [e] for power supply.

TABLE 10.5. *Environmental requirements*[a]

Total Heat Dissipation
    Permanent magnet 0[c]
    Resistive system 350,000 BTU/hr[b]
    Superconducting (S/C) system
        100,000 BTU/hr
Altitude[c] (max)
    6000 ft (1828 m)
Ambient temperature range
    +60°F to +75°F (+15°C to 24°C)
    Field uniformity of permanent magnet
        may be very heat sensitive
Helium venting (S/C system only)
    Normal range −375 liters/hr
    During quench −1.5 × 10[5] liters

Source: General Electric.
[a] Expected maximum values.
[b] Includes about 200,000 BTU/hr, which is removed from magnet room by cooling water.
[c] Not applicable to permanent magnet.

It should be noted in the floor plan that exit from the NMR magnet should allow for rapid straight line patient removal from the NMR suite to an area where patient monitoring and life-support equipment will operate satisfactorily in case of a medical emergency. Although

TABLE 10.6. *Power requirements*

Permanent magnet
    Suite power requirements, 40 KW
    (With the permanent magnet, there is no quenching nor any special power requirements. There is a minimal fringe field and limited missile effect, so site selection is relatively simple by comparison. There are no costly cryogenic expenses and there are no moving parts except for the motorized patient bed.)

Resistive system
    Max. power: 150 KVA
    Voltage: 480 volts, 3 phase, 50/80 Hz
    Voltage tolerance: +10%, −15%
    Current (total at 480 volts): Momentary 357 amp
                          Continuous 312 amp

Superconducting system
    Max. power: 70 KVA
    Voltage: 480 volts, 3 phase, 50/60 Hz
    Voltage tolerance: +10%, −15%
    Current (total at 480 volts): Momentary 175 amp
                          Continuous 146 amp

Sources: General Electric, Siemens, and Fonar.

not listed on the diagram, RF shielding is necessary, and for most sites at least a 90 db reduction is required. In addition, reinforcement of the floor is necessary for these systems with a maximum loading of 10,000 kg.

With so many computers, terminals, image intensifiers, and other CRTs in and around most hospitals and offices, the effects of magnetic fields on these devices are terribly important to evaluate. One useful approach is a measure of the anisotropy—that is, unequal distortions in two dimensions of the susceptible components of the CRT (i.e., unequal distortions of the CRT image). In general, the effects are slightly greater on black-and-white than on color CRTs, but an unshielded system can expect about 2% anisotropy; however, iron shielding will decrease the effect.

Table 10.4 lists some magnet specifications for several types of NMR systems. Tables 10.5 and 10.6 lists environmental and power requirements, respectively.

Chapter 11

Nuclear Magnetic Resonance Review Quiz

Readers who now feel they have a basic understanding of magnetic resonance principles should take the following quiz. If you are comfortable with the material and answer the majority of the questions correctly, the quiz can serve as a quick review of NMR and indicate those sections of the text that should be reviewed in the future.

1. When an oscillating compass needle is brought closer to a bar magnet, the frequency of oscillation:
   A. decreases
   B. stays the same
   C. increases
   D. all of the above depending on conditions
2. The magnetic field strength of the earth versus the magnetic field strength of a typical magnetic resonance scanner is:
   A. 0.5/2000 Larmor
   B. 0.5/2000 G
   C. 2/1000 Fourier
   D. 2/1000 G
3. T_1 and T_2 are two decay constants associated with NMR imaging. Which of the following is true of these constants?
   A. T_1 is equal to 2 T_2
   B. T_1 is less than or equal to T_2
   C. T_1 is greater than or equal to T_2
   D. 2 T_1 equals T_2
4. NMR imaging depends on the interaction of:
   A. magnetic fields and X-rays
   B. magnetic fields and radio waves
   C. electromagnetic waves and electric fields
   D. electromagnetic waves and radio waves

5. The Larmor (resonant) frequency, ω, is determined by:
   A. the magnetic field strength
   B. the nuclear decay constant
   C. the magnetogyric ratio
   D. the magnetogyric ratio and magnetic field strength
6. For hydrogen (protons, ^1H) placed in a 0.1 T (1000 G) field, the resonant frequency will be:
   A. 0.98 MHz
   B. 4.26 MHz
   C. 6.39 MHz
   D. 0.65 MHz
7. What is resonating in NMR imaging?
   A. the sample atoms
   B. the sample molecules
   C. biopolymers larger than 40,000 molecular weight
8. The purpose of the gradient magnetic field coils is to:
   A. direct the flow of protons
   B. excite the emission of radio wave photons
   C. provide spatial localization of NMR emissions
   D. cause emission of radio wave photons
9. In comparison to other techniques such as CT and radiography, the most important characteristic of NMR imaging is:
   A. improved cost
   B. improved contrast resolution
   C. improved spatial resolution
   D. improved speed
10. Magnetic resonance is a phenomenon that occurs when a static external magnetic field is applied to a tissue and occurs in all atoms with:
    A. protons
    B. electrons
    C. neutrons
    D. unpaired protons, electrons or neutrons

Now review the answers and then review the test in those areas where you feel your understanding of the topic requires it.

Answers to NMR quiz:
1. C   4. B   7. A   10. D
2. B   5. D   8. C
3. B   6. B   9. B

Glossary

Absorption line. A relative peak in the frequency spectrum from NMR spectroscopy that corresponds to a characteristic absorption of the radio frequency (RF pulse).

Adiabatic fast passage. A technique used to invert net tissue magnetization by sweeping the magnetic field (or RF spectrum) through the resonant frequency.

American College of Radiology Imaging Terms. See pulse sequence, Interpulse time, Repetition time (TR), Inversion time (T_I), and Echo Time (TE).

Angular frequency (ω). Rotational frequency usually expressed in hertz (Hz). Nuclear particles spin around a central axis. The measure of this rotational motion is called *angular momentum*. Other atomic particles, especially electrons, may also possess orbital angular momentum as well as spin angular momentum.

Chemical shift. In NMR spectroscopy chemical shifts are observable as slightly displaced resonant peaks in higher resolution (field homogeneity 1/10^6) NMR systems and result from the differential shielding effect of electrons orbiting in the molecule. (These chemical shifts, in other words, are due to the regional magnetic forces within the molecular environment.)

Coherence. Used in NMR to describe the magnetic moments of nuclear particles that are rotating or precessing in phase.

Diamagnetic. Pertains to a sample in which the internal and induced magnetic field is in the opposite direction to and usually much weaker than the external magnetic field.

Echo time (TE). Time between middle of 90° pulse and middle of spin echo production. For multiple echoes use TE1, TE2, etc.

Fast Fourier transformation (FFT). A fast and efficient algorithm for calculating Fourier transform analyses on a digital computer.

Fourier transformation (FT). A mathematical algorithm that is capable of converting complex wave forms into either a signal that is observable as an amplitude versus time or a signal of amplitude versus frequency. The process is a representation of the complex wave function by a sum of sine and cosine. The FFT is a somewhat shortened version of the longer FT.

Gauss. A unit of magnetic field strength or magnetic flux density. NMR magnetic field strengths expressed in this system are usually expressed as kilogauss (10^3 G).

Gradient magnetic field. A magnetic field whose strength varies along a linear direction.

Gyromagnetic ratio (γ). This is a parameter relating the nuclear magnetic frequency to the static magnetic field strength, and it is characteristic or specific for each particular nuclear species. It is also called the *magnetogyric* and is defined by the Larmor equation.

Hertz (Hz). The unit of frequency measurement indicating the number of complete cycles completed in one second.

Image acquisition time. To calculate acquisition time: Total acquisition time = (TR) × (acquisition matrix) × (2) × (no. of signal averages) × no. of slices.

Interpulse times. Times between successive RF pulses used in pulse sequences. Particularly important are the inversion time (T1) in inversion recovery and the time between a 90° pulse and subsequent 180° pulse to produce a spin echo. This interval will be approximately one half the spin echo time (TE). The time between repetitions of pulse sequences is the repetition time (TR).

Inversion recovery. An imaging sequence involving an 180° to 90° RF pulse sequence that provides T1 discrimination.

Inversion time (T1). Time between middle of inverting RF pulse and middle of subsequent 90° pulse to detect amount of longitudinal magnetization.

Larmor relation. Larmor frequency is the resonant frequency in a given magnetic field where the relationship for hydrogen is 42.58 MHz/T.

Lorentzian line. A radio-frequency absorption line obtained from a spectroscopy experiment with a narrow peak and long tails.

Magnetic dipole. Essentially a bar magnetic or any north and south magnetic poles that are separated by some distance. Spinning charged particles can create magnetic dipole moments.

Magnetic moment. The torque or force exerted in a magnetic field of given strength when the axis of the magnet is at right angles to the field. Nuclear magnetic moment is the magnetic moment associated with spinning charged nuclear particles.

Magnetization. In NMR imaging magnetization generally refers to net tissue magnetization, which is the net effect of the ensemble or large numbers of protons, a slight majority of which are oriented parallel to the static magnetic field. It is this slight excess of parallel protons that confer net tissue magnetization to the tissue or sample being scanned.

Nuclear magnetic resonance (NMR). The resonant emission and absorption of radio-frequency electromagnetic energy by nuclei in a static external magnetic field. The resonant frequency of absorption is directly proportional to the strength of the external field.

Paramagnetic. Pertains to a sample in which the internal induced magnetic field is in the same direction as the applied external field. This property, however, is not retained when the external field is removed.

Paramagnetic atoms. Atoms that slightly increase a magnetic field when they are placed within it are referred to as paramagnetic. They, in general, have an odd number of electrons with a partially filled inner electron shell.

Precession (wobbling). A spinning top in the earth's gravitational field or a proton in an external magnetic field wobble or precess around their axis.

The frequency of precession ω in NMR scanning is given by the Larmor equation $\omega = \gamma B$, where γ is the gyromagnetic ratio and B is the static magnetic field.

Probe. In an NMR spectroscopy system, the part that contains the sample and the radio frequency (RF coil) is referred to as the probe.

Pulse sequences. Sets of RF (and/or gradient) magnetic field pulses and time spacings between these pulses; used in conjunction with gradient magnetic fields and NMR signal reception to produce NMR images.

Quenching. Loss (usually unexpected) of the near absolute zero temperatures induced by the surrounding liquid helium in a superconducting magnet. When superconductivity is lost, the magnet will acutely become resistive.

Radio frequency (RF). The portion of the electromagnetic spectrum containing the radio waves with wavelengths between 10 and 10^4 m and 10^4 to 10^9 Hz.

Radio frequency (RF coil). The antenna used for transmitting or irradiating radio-frequency pulses and receiving the emitted signal in NMR imaging systems.

Radio frequency (RF pulse). The radio frequency—usually of short duration–generated by an RF oscillator and transmitted by an RF coil.

Relaxation. The process by which molecules move between high-energy and low-energy states. The method of relaxation depends on the physical state of the tissue or specimen being studied. In NMR it is the time required for magnetization to return to equilibrium after an RF pulse.

Repetition time (TR). The period of time between the beginning of a pulse sequence and the beginning of a succeeding (essentially identical) pulse sequence.

Resonance. The exchange of energy at specified frequencies. In NMR it is the process by which nuclei absorb radio-frequency energy that causes the protons to flip between upper and lower or parallel and antiparallel energy states.

Rotating frame. A concept originally applied by Tesla in which a frame of reference rotates with the precessing nuclear moments. In this system the motion of the precessing magnetization is in some respects easier to describe.

Shim coils. Flat wire coils used to produce small magnetic gradients in an NMR system to correct field inhomogeneities. These are used extensively in fitting magnets into structures that were not designed for NMR systems.

Signal-to-noise. In NMR image, noise increases in the coil as the square root of the frequency; however, the nuclear signal increases as the frequency squared. The ideal signal-to-noise ratio is proportional to $f^{3/2}$. Theoretically, at higher field strengths, this relationship was thought to have changed because of the increased radio-frequency absorption that was due to the electrical conductivity of the body. Recently, however, experiments have shown that proton imaging can be performed at 1.5 T and many of these theoretical concerns may not have practical consequences.

Spectrum. The spectrum in NMR is the display of the relative radio-frequency absorption peaks in the frequency domain plotted as a function of their resonant frequencies.

Spin. A property of a spinning particle, electron, neutron, or proton that determines its magnetic moment. The spin of an electron or proton is one-half.

Spin-echo. An NMR signal that occurs at fixed intervals after a perturbation and results from phase coherence. The signal has a crescendo-decrescendo character and is called the *echo* or *spin-echo* signal.

T_1 *relaxation time.* Also called *spin-lattice* or *longitudinal relaxation time*. This is the exponential time constant at which the component of magnetization parallel to the external field returns to equilibrium conditions. This decay results from the interaction of a nucleus (spin) with its physical surroundings (lattice) and is therefore called spin-lattice relaxation.

T_2 *relaxation time.* Also called *spin-spin* or *transverse relaxation time*. It is the exponential time consonant that the component of magnetization, which is perpendicular to the external field, requires to return to equilibrium conditions in a homogeneous magnetic field. It results from the decay of coherence in the perpendicular plane and is the result of interactions of the spinning nuclei with the spin of identical nuclei pointing in the opposite direction and hence is called spin-spin relaxation.

T2*. Effective transverse relaxation time in a nonhomogeneous field ($T2* < T_2$).

Tesla. The usual unit of magnetic field strength that is equal to 10,000 G.

Three-dimensional and two-dimensional Fourier transform (2DFT and 3DFT). An imaging technique in which spatial information is phase encoded in the precessing nuclei by the selective use of gradient magnetic fields.

Zeugmatography. A term originally used by Lauterbur taken from the Greek root *zeugma* meaning "to join together." This word was chosen to indicate the use of electromagnetic waves and nuclear magnetic resonance as the yoke between the two forms of energy in this type of imaging.

References

1. Abragam, A. (1961): *Principles of Nuclear Magnetism*. Clarendon Press, Oxford.
2. Ackerman, J. J. H., Grove, T. H., Wong, G. G., Gadian, D. G., and Radda, G. K. (1980): Mapping of metabolites in whole animals by 31P NMR using surface coils. *Nature,* 283:167–170.
3. Alfidi, R. J., Haaga, J. R., Yousef, S. J., Bryan, P. J., Fletcher, B. D., LiPuma, J. P., Morrison, S. C., Kaufman, B., Richey, J. B., Hinshaw, W. S., Kramer, D. M., Yeung, N. Y., Cohen, A. M., Butler, H. E., Ament, A. E., and Lieberman, J. M. (1982): Preliminary experimental results in humans and animals with a superconducting whole-body, nuclear magnetic resonance scanner. *Radiology,* 143:175–186.
4. Alfidi, R. J., Haaga, J. R., El Yousef, S. J., Bryan, P. J., et al. (1982): Preliminary experimental results in animals with a superconducting, whole body nuclear magnetic resonance scanner. *Radiology,* 143:179–181.
5. Andrew, E. R. (1969): *Nuclear Magnetic Resonance*. Cambridge University Press, Cambridge.
6. Batnitzky, S., Price, H. I., Cook, P. N., Cook, L. T., and Dwyer, S. J. III (1981): Three-dimensional computer reconstruction from surface contours for head CT examinations. *J. Comp. Assist. Tomogr.,* 5:60–67.
7. Becker, E. D. (1980): *High Resolution NMR—Theory and Chemical Applications,* 2nd edition. Academic Press, New York.
8. Bloch, F. (1946): Nuclear induction. *Phys. Rev.* 70:nos. 7, 8.
9. Bloch, F., Hansen, W. W., and Packard, M. E. (1946): Nuclear induction. *Phys. Rev.,* 69:127.
10. Bradley, W. G. (1982): *NMR Tomography*. Diasonics Interactive Education Program.
11. Brady, T. J., Goldman, M. R., Pykett, I. L., Buonanno, F. S., Kistler, J. P., Newhouse, J. H., Burt, C. T., Hinshaw, W. S., and Pohost, G. M. (1982): Proton nuclear magnetic resonance imaging of regionally ischemic cannine hearts: effect of paramagnetic proton signal enhancement. *Radiology,* 144: 343–347.
12. Brasch, R. C., Nitecki, D. E., London, D., Tozer, T. N., Doemey, J., Tuck, L. D., and Wolff, S. (1983): Evaluation of nitroxide stable free radicals for contrast enhancement in NMR Imaging. *J. Magn. Reson. (in press)*.
13. Brunner, P., and Ernest, R. R. (1979): Sensitivity and performance time in NMR imaging. *J. Magn. Reson.,* 33:83–106, 1979.
14. Budinger, T. F. (1983): Hazards from D.C. and A.C. magnetic fields. *J. Magn. Reson. (in press)*.
15. Budinger, T. F. (1981): Nuclear magnetic resonance (NMR in vivo studies: known thresholds for health effects). *J. Comput. Assist. Tomogr.,* 5:800–811.
16. Burnett, J. L., and Know, F. G. (1980): Renal interstitial pressure and sodium excretion during renal vein construction. *Am. J. Physiol.,* 238:F279–F282.
17. Carr, H. Y., and Purcell, E. M. (1954): Effects of diffusion on free precession in nuclear resonance experiments. *Phys. Rev.,* 94:no. 3.
18. Carrington, A., and McLachlanad (1967): *Introduction to Magnetic Resonance*. Harper & Row, New York.
19. Chan, L., French, M. E., Gadian, D. G., Morris, P. J., Radda, G. K., Bore, P. J., Ross, B. D., and Styles, P. (1983): Study of human kidneys prior to transplantation by phosphorus nuclear magnetic resonance. In: *Organ Transplantation III*. edited by D. E. Pegg, I. Jacobson, and N. A. Halasz. MTP Press, Ltd. *(in press)*.

20. Cohen, S. M., Shulman, R. G., and McLaughlin, A. C. (1979): Effects of ethanol on alanine metabolism in perfused mouse liver studied by ^{13}C NMR. *Proc. Natl. Acad. Sci. (USA)*, 76:4808–4812.

21. Crooks, L., Arakawa, M., Hoenninger, J., Watts, J., McRee, R., Kaufman, L., Davis, P. L., Margulis, A. R., and DeGroot, J. (1982): Nuclear magnetic resonance whole-body imager operating at 3.5 K gauss. *Radiology*, 143:169–181.

22. Crooks, L., Sheldon, P., Kaufman, L., Rowan, W., and Miller, T. (1982): Quantification of obstruction in vessels by nuclear magnetic resonance. *IEEE Trans. Nucl. Sci. NS-29*, 3:1181–1185.

23. Crooks, L. E., Arakawa, M., Hoenninger, J., Watts, J., McRee, R., Kaufman, L., Davis, P. L., and Margulis, A. R. (1982): NMR whole body imager operating at 3.5 K. gauss. *Radiology*, 143:169–174.

24. Crooks, L. E., Mills, C. M., Davis, P. L., Brant-Zawadski, M., Hoenninger, J., Arakawa, M., Watts, J., and Kaufman, L. (1983): The effects of imaging parameters on contrast. *Radiology (in press)*.

25. Damadian, R. (1971): Tumor detection by nuclear magnetic resonance. *Science*, 171:1151–1153.

26. Damadian, R., Goldsmith, M., and Minhoff, L. (1977): NMR in cancer: XVI Fonar image of the live human body. *Physiol. Chem. Phys.*, 9.

27. Davis, P. L., Kaufman, L., Crooks, L. E., and Miller, T. R. (1981): Detectability of hepatomas in rat livers by nuclear magnetic resonance imaging. *Invest. Radiol.* 16:354–359.

28. Doyle, F. H., Gore, J. C., and Pennock, J. M. (1981): Relaxation rate enhancement observed in vivo by NMR imaging. *J. Comp. Assist. Tomogr.*, 5:295–296.

29. Doyle, F. H., Pennock, J. M., Banks, L. M., McDonnell, M. J., Bydder, G. M., Steiner, R. E., Young, I. R., Clark, G. J., Pasmore, T., and Gilderdale, D. J. (1982): Nuclear magnetic resonance imaging of the liver: initial experience. *AJR* 138:193–200.

30. Fuchs, H., Pizer, S. M., Cohen, J. S., and Brooks, F. P., Jr. (1979): A three-dimensional display for medical images from slices. *Les Collogfues de l'Inserim*, 88:581–602.

31. Fullerton, G. D. (1982): Basic concepts for nuclear magnetic resonance imaging, *Magn. Reson. Imag.*, 1:39–55.

32. Gadian, D. G. (1982): *Nuclear Magnetic Resonance and Its Applications to Living Systems*. Oxford University Press, Oxford.

33. Gadian, D. G., and Radda, G. K. (1983): NMR spectroscopy: in vivo and in vitro medical studies. *J. Magn. Reson. (in press)*.

34. Gadian, D. G., and Radda, G. K. (1981): NMR studies of tissue metabolism. *Ann. Ren. Biochem.*, 50:69–83.

35. Gadian, D. G., Radda, G. K., Brown, T. R., Chance, E., Dawson, M. J., and Wilkie, D. R. (1981): The activity of creatine kinase in frog skeletal muscle studied by saturation-transfer nuclear magnetic resonance. *Biochem. J.*, 194:215–228.

36. Gadian, D. G., Radda, G. K., Ross, B. D., Hockaday, J., Bore, P. J., Taylor, D. J., and Styles, P. (1981): Examination of a myopathy by phosphorus nuclear magnetic resonance. *Lancet*, 2:774–775.

37. Goldman, M. R., Brady, T. J., Pykett, I. L., Burt, C. T., Newhouse, J. H., Buonanno, F., Kistler, P., Hinshaw, W., and Pohost, G. (1981): Cardiac application of nuclear magnetic resonance imaging. In: *Bowman Gray Symposium on Nuclear Magnetic Resonance Imaging*, pp. 171–173. Bowman Gray School of Medicine Press, Winston-Salem, North Carolina.

38. Goldman, M. R., Pykett, I. L., Brady, T. J., and Pohost, G. M. (1983): Gated

proton NMR imaging in dogs with experimental myocardial infarction. *J. Magn. Reson. (in press)*.

39. Gordon, R. E., Hanley, P. E., Shaw, D., Gadian, D. G., Radda, G. K., Styles, P., Bore, P. H., and Chan, L. (1980): Localization of metabolites in animals using 31P topical magnetic resonance. *Nature* 287:736–738.
40. Harris, L. D. (1981): Identification of the optimal orientation of oblique sections through multiple parallel CT sections. *J. Comp. Assist. Tomogr.*, 5:881–887.
41. Harris, L. D., Robb, R. A., Yuen, T. S., and Ritman, E. L. (1979): Display and visualization of three-dimensional reconstructed anatomic morphology: experience with the thorax, heart, and coronary vasculature of dogs. *J. Comp. Assist. Tomgr.*, 3:439–446.
42. Hawkes, R. C., Holland, G. N., Moore, W. S., Roebuck, E. J., and Worthington, B. S. (1981): NMR tomography of the normal heart. *J. Comp. Assist. Tomogr.*, 5:605–612.
43. Heidelberger, E., and Lauterbur, P. C. (1983): Gas phase ^{19}F-NMR zeugmatography: a new approach to lung ventilation imaging. *J. Magn. Reson. (in press)*.
44. Heidelberger, E., Petersen, S. B., and Lauterbur, P. C. (1983): 3D synchronized proton NMR imaging of the beating heart. *J. Magn. Reson. (in press)*.
45. Herman, G. T., and Udapa, J. K. (1981): Display 3-D discrete surfaces. *Proceed. Soc. Phot. Instr. Eng.*, 283:90–97.
46. Hollis, D. P., Nunnally, R. L., Taylor, G. J., Weisfeldt, M. L., and Jacobus, W. E. (1978): Phosphorus NMR studies of heart physiology. *J. Magn. Reson.*, 29:319–330.
47. Hoult, D. I., Busby, S. J. W., Gadian, D. G., Radda, G., Richards, R. E., and Seeley, P. J. (1974): Observation of tissue metabolites using 31P nuclear magnetic resonance. *Nature*, 252:285–287.
47a. Jardetzky, O., and Wertz, J. P. (1956): Detection of sodium complexes by nuclear spin resonance. *Am. J. Physiol.*, 187:608.
48. Karstaedt, N., Witcofski, R. L., and Partain, C. L., editors (1982): *Proceedings of an International Symposium on NMR imaging*. Bowman Gray School of Medicine Press, Winston-Salem, North Carolina.
49. Kaufman, L., Crooks, L., and Margulis, A. R., editors (1981): *Nuclear Magnetic Resonance Imaging in Medicine*. Igaku-Shoin, New York.
50. Kiricuta, I. C., Jr., and Simplaceanu, V. (1975): Tissue water content and nuclear magnetic resonance in normal and tumor tissues. *Cancer Res.*, 35:1164–1167.
51. Kumar, A., Welti, D., and Ernst, R. R. (1975): NMR Fourier zeugmatography. *J. Magn. Reson.*, 18:69–83.
52. Lang, J., Sances, A., Jr., and Larson, S. J. (1969): Determination of specific cerebral impedance and cerebral current density during the application of diffuse electrical currents. *Med. Biol. Eng.*, 7:517–526.
53. Lauterbur, P. C. (1973): Image formation by induced local interactions: examples employing nuclear magnetic resonance. *Nature*, 242–5394:190.
54. Lovsund, P., Nilsson, S. E. G., Reuter, T., and Oberg, P. (1980): Magnetophosphenes: a quantitative analysis of thresholds. *Med. Biol. Eng. Comput.*, 18:326–334.
55. Luiten, A. L., Uijen, C. V., Locher, P. R., Boef, J. D., Dijk, P. V., and Holzschere, C. (1983): Optimization at the 1st annual meeting of the society of magnetic resonance in medicine. *J. Magn. Reson. (in press)*.
56. Mansfield, P. (1981): Critical evaluation of NMR imaging techniques. *Proc. of ISNMRI*, 81–87.
57. Mansfield, P. (1977): Multi-planar image formation using NMR spin echoes. *J. Phys. C.: Solid State Phys.*, 10.

58. Mansfield, P., and Morris, P. G. (1982): *NMR Imaging in Biomedicine,* pp. 155–201. Academic Press, New York.
59. Mansfield, P., and Moris, P. G. (1982): In: *Advances in Magnetic Resonance, Special Suppl. 2: NMR Imaging in Biomedicine,* edited by J. S. Waugh. Academic Press, New York.
60. Mansfield, P., Ordidge, R. J., Rzedzian, R. R., Doyle, M., and Guilfoyle, D. (1983): Real-time dynamic imaging by NMR. *J. Magn. Reson. (in press).*
61. Marchandise, X., Graff, R., Epstein, F., Pike, M., Brezis, P., Silva, J., Ingwall, J., DeLayre, J., and Fossel, E. (1983): NA-23 NMR observation of intra and extracellular sodium in the isolated perfused rat kidney. *J. Magn. Reson. (in press).*
62. Matthews, P. M., Bland, J. L., Gadian, D. G., and Radda, G. K. (1981): The steady-state rate of ATP synthesis in the perfused rat heart measured by 31P NMR saturation transfer. *Biochem. Biophys. Res. Commun.,* 103:1052–1059.
63. Maudsley, A. A., Hilal, S. K., Simon, H. E., and Perman, W. H. (1983): Multinuclear NMR imaging. *J. Magn. Reson. (in press).*
64. McConnel, H. M. (1976): Molecular motion in biological membranes. In: *Spin Labeling, Theory and Applications,* edited by L. J. Berlinear. Academic Press, New York.
65. Neidinger, J. W., and Deutsch, S. (1971): Control and measurement of current density distribution in the brain. In: *Neuroelectric Research,* edited by D. V. Reynolds and A. E. Sjoberg. Charles C Thomas, Springfield, Illinois.
66. Newman, R. J., Bore, P. J., Chan, L., Gadian, D. G., Styles, P., Taylor, D. J., and Radda, G. K. (1982): Nuclear magnetic resonance studies of forearm muscle in Duchenne dystrophy. *Br. Med. J.,* 284:1072–1074.
67. Nunnally, R. L., and Peshock, R. W. (1983): In vivo and in situ metabolic evaluations by C-13 and P-31 NMR. *J. Magn. Reson. (in press).*
68. Oldendorf, W. H. (1982): NMR imaging: its potential clinical impact. *Hosp. Prac.,* 114–124.
69. Oldendorf, W. H. (1980): *The Quest for an Image of Brain.* Raven Press, New York.
70. Ordidge, R. J., Mansfield, P., Doyle, M., and Coupland, R. E. (1982): Real-time moving images by NMR. *Radiology,* 142:244.
71. Partain, C. L., James, A. E., Rollo, F. D., and Price, R. R. (1983): *Nuclear Magnetic Resonance (NMR) Imaging.* W. B. Saunders, Philadelphia.
72. Purcell, E. M., Taurry, H. C., and Pound, R. V. (1946): Resonance absorption by nuclear magnetic moments in a solid. *Phys. Rev.,* 69:37.
73. Pykett, I. L. (1982): NMR imaging in medicine. *Sci. Am.,* 246:78–88.
74. Pykett, I. L., Newhouse, J. H., Buonanno, F. S., Brady, T. J., Goldman, M. R., Kistler, J. P., and Pohost, G. M. (1982): Principles of nuclear magnetic resonance imaging. *Radiology,* 143:157–168.
75. Radda, G. K., Bore, P. J., Gadian, D. G., Ross, B. D., Stles, U., Taylor, D. J., and Morgan-Hughes, J. (1982): 31P NMR examination of two patients with NADH- CoQ reductase deficiency. *Nature,* 295:608–609.
76. Ross, B. D., Radda, G. K., Gadian, D. G., Rocker, G., Esiri, M., and Falconer-Smith, J. (1981): Examination of a case of suspected McArlde's syndrome by 31P nuclear magnetic resonance. *N. Eng. J. Med.,* 304:1338–1342.
77. Roy, O. Z. (1980): Technical note: summary of cardiac fibrillation thresholds for 60 Hz currents and voltages applied directly to the heart. *Med. Biol. Eng. Comput.,* 18:657–659.
78. Schwartz, J. L., and Crooks, L. E. (1982): NMR imaging produces no observable mutations or cytotoxicity in mammalian cells. *AJR,* 139:583–585.
79. Shoubridge, E. A., Briggs, R. W., and Radda, G. K. (1982): 31P NMR saturation

transfer measurements of the steady state rates of creatine kinase and ATP synthetase in the rat brain. *Febs. Lett.,* 140:288–292.

80. Singer, J. R. (1978): Nuclear magnetic resonance diffusion and flow measurements and an introduction to spin phase graphing. *J. Phys. E. Sci. Instr.,* 2.

81. Smith, F. W., Mallard, J. R., Reid, A., and Hutchinson, J. M. S. (1981): Nuclear magnetic resonance tomography imaging in liver disease. *Lancet,* 1:963–966.

82. Sutherland, R. J., Hutchinson, J. M. S. (1973): Magnetic resonance zeugmatography. *Nature (Lond.),* 242:190.

83. Taylor, D. J., Bore, P. J., Styles, P., Gadian, D. G., Radda, G. K. (1983): 31P NMR studies of normal human muscle. (*Submitted.*)

84. Wyrwicz, A., Schofield, J., Burt, C. T. (1981): Multinuclear NMR studies of blood in a flowing system. In: *Non-invasive Probes of Tissue Metabolism.* edited by J. Cohen, pp. 149–171. John Wiley and Sons, New York.

85. Young, I. R., Bailes, D. R., Burl, M., Collins, A. G., Smith, D. T., McDonnel, M. R., Orr, J. S., Banks, L. M., Bydder, G. M., Greenspan, R. H., and Steiner, R. E. (1982): Initial clinical evaluation of a whole body nuclear magnetic resonance (NMR) tomograph. *J. Comp. Assist. Tomogr.,* 6:1–18.

Appendix I

Schematic representation of RF excitation and emission sequence.

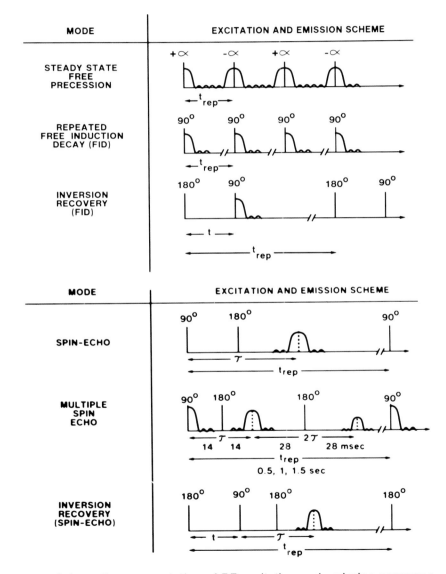

FIG. 1. Schematic representation of RF excitation and emission sequence.

Appendix II

Schematic representation and figure of a typical imaging system that show the six basic subsystems: gradient, magnet, radio, computer, data storage, and display.

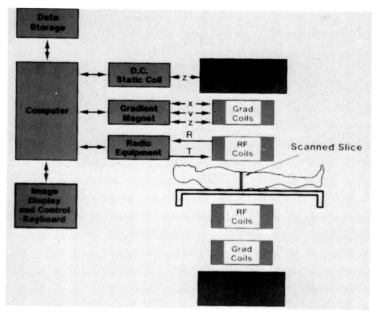

FIG. 1. Schematic representation of typical NMR imaging system.

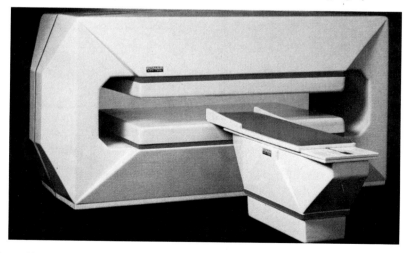

FIG. 2. NMR scanner—permanent magnet. Copyright Fonar Corporation. Image provided courtesy of Fonar Corporation.

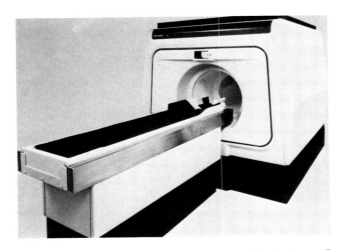

FIG. 3. NMR scanner—resistive magnet. (Copyright Technicare Corporation. NMR image provided by courtesy of Technicare Corporation and the Cleveland Clinic Foundation.)

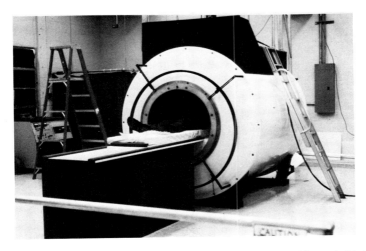

FIG. 4. NMR scanner—superconduction magnet system. (Copyright General Electric Company. NMR image provided by courtesy of The General Electric Company.)

Appendix III

American College of Radiology Imaging Definitions

Partial saturation

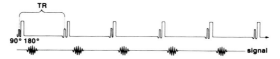

Sequence illustrated with 0.2 S TR (approximately 7 msec elapses between the 90° and 180° pulses)

Inversion recovery

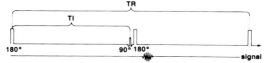

Sequence illustrated with 1.0 S TR and 500 msec TI

Spin echo

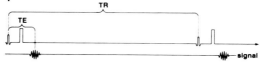

Sequence illustrated with 0.8 S TR and 100 msec TE (approximately 50 ms elapses between the 90° and 180° pulses)

Multiple echo

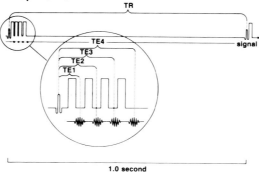

Sequence illustrated with 1.0 S TR and TE of 25, 50, 75 and 100 msec.

FIG. 1. Repetition time (TR). The period of time between the beginning of a pulse sequence and the beginning of a succeeding (essentially identical) pulse sequence. Inversion time (T_1). Time between middle of inverting RF pulse and middle of subsequent 90° pulse to detect amount of longitudinal magnetization. Echo time (TE). Time between middle of 90° pulse and middle of spin echo production. For multiple echoes use TE1, TE2, etc. (Courtesy of General Electric Co.)

Subject Index